# THE
# BRAIN BOOST
# DIET PLAN

# THE
# BRAIN BOOST
## DIET PLAN

4 weeks to optimize your mood, memory and brain health for life

Christine Bailey

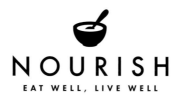

# NOURISH
### EAT WELL, LIVE WELL

# THE **BRAIN BOOST** DIET PLAN

Christine Bailey

First published in the UK and USA in 2018 by
Nourish, an imprint of Watkins Media Limited
19 Cecil Court
London WC2N 4EZ
enquiries@nourishbooks.com

Managing Editor: Kate Fox
Editor: Jan Cutler
Designer: Karen Smith
Production: Uzma Taj
Photography: Toby Scott
Food Stylist: Rebecca Woods
Prop Stylist: Linda Berlin

A CIP record for this book is available from the
British Library

ISBN: 9781848993396

10 9 8 7 6 5 4 3 2 1

Colour reproduction by XY Digital
Printed in China

**Publisher's note**
While every care has been taken in compiling the
recipes for this book, Watkins Media Limited, or any
other persons who have been involved in working on
this publication, cannot accept responsibility for any
errors or omissions, inadvertent or not, that may be
found in the recipes or text, nor for any problems that
may arise as a result of preparing one of these recipes.
If you are pregnant or breastfeeding or have any
special dietary requirements or medical conditions, it
is advisable to consult a medical professional before
following any of the recipes contained in this book.

**Notes on the recipes**
Unless otherwise stated:
• Always use filtered water, if possible, when making
  fermented foods
• Use organic ingredients and animal products, such as
  gelatine, from grass-fed animals, where possible
• Use medium fruit and vegetables
• Use medium (US large) organic or free-range eggs
• Use fresh herbs, spices and chillies
• Use granulated sugar (Americans can use ordinary
  granulated sugar when caster sugar is specified)
• Do not mix metric, imperial and US cup
  measurements
• 1 tsp = 5ml  1 tbsp = 15ml  1 cup = 240ml

nourishbooks.com

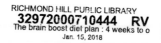

# CONTENTS

How's your brain health?                    6
How to use this book                       10

**WEEK 1:** Cleanse                        12
**WEEK 2:** Renew                          28
**WEEK 3:** Protect                        36
**WEEK 4:** Revitalize                     42

The Brain Boost Diet Plan                  50
Meal Plans                                 56

## RECIPES

Your Basic Pantry                          60
Breakfasts                                 76
Soups & Salads                            104
Main Meals                                132
Desserts & Snacks                         182

Index                                     212

# How's your brain health?

**Are you worried about losing your memory? Do you find it hard to concentrate and focus on tasks? Do you struggle with brain fog, low mood or depression? If so, now is the time to take action. Our modern diet and lifestyle can take its toll on the brain. Degeneration can affect people of all ages, and begins decades before symptoms become evident.**

Our mood, our memory and our ability to think clearly are all very much dependent on the functioning of our brain cells and the production of brain chemicals. A decline in mental ability, mood or capacity for learning is not inevitable as we age, however. Our brain can actually thrive at any age through specific dietary choices and lifestyle habits.

The Brain Boost Diet will show you how to nourish your brain by following my revolutionary four-week programme, which includes recipes for each stage. It is based on the latest research into maintaining brain health, boosting mood and keeping the mind sharp.

## My story

Twenty years ago I watched my grandmother disappear from me day by day, as Alzheimer's took over. The cruellest of diseases and perhaps the most dreaded of brain disorders, Alzheimer's robbed her of the last five years of her life and left the family feeling hopeless and devastated.

Since then I have researched extensively and worked with numerous clients who are struggling with myriad brain-health disorders – ranging from ADHD (attention deficit disorder), low mood and depression, addictions, headaches, migraines, anxiety, dementia or difficulty performing to capacity. These conditions affect people of all ages and backgrounds. In addition, if there's one health concern that seems to affect most people as they get older, it's how to keep the brain sharp and avoid dementia in any form. I have therefore spent years researching, working alongside experts involved in functional medicine and supporting clients to develop dietary strategies, recipes and programmes to nourish the brain.

## WHAT WE EAT MATTERS

Our typical Western diet does not support a healthy brain – in fact, it destroys it. This might sound extreme, but our obsession with processed and convenience foods, grains, carbohydrates and sugar are the exact foods that will accelerate our body's ageing process – and that includes our brain. It might surprise you that having type-2 diabetes doubles your risk of Alzheimer's disease, but the two conditions are connected through their shared problem of a poor diet, and how eating processed foods, refined carbohydrates, gluten grains and sugar in all its forms is poisoning your brain.

## Boost your brain the smart way

My four-week programme will help you to make positive changes to your brain health, by showing you how to detox your brain, ditch the sugar and grains and, in their place, nourish your brain with healthy fats, protein and plants.

What makes this programme unique is that it looks at the underlying factors contributing to poor brain health and addresses each one week by week. The programme also focuses on the health of another very vital organ for a healthy brain – and that is our gut. If you have ever had stomach or digestive problems, it is likely due to your gut health. I will show you the importance of the gut–brain link in influencing how we think and feel, our overal energy and vitality, and, more importantly, how the daily dietary choices we make impact our gut health.

## "WHY ISN'T MY BRAIN WORKING?"

The brain is the most complex organ in our body. With a weight of 1.3kg/3lb it is one of our heaviest organs, demanding the most oxygen and glucose, and using about 30 per cent of the body's glucose to function. In a healthy brain, information from one neuron (brain cell) flows to another neuron across a small gap that separates them, called a synapse. In a healthy brain, the neurons are stimulated, creating branches like the roots of a plant into one another. This enhances communication between the brain cells and facilitates better brain function. This ability to build pathways in the brain is known as plasticity and it enables you to develop mental processes, such as learning new skills and information.

## The failing brain

A sign that neurons are being lost more rapidly is poor plasticity; for example, you might be finding it harder to learn new information than you used to. As we age it is not inevitable that plasticity declines, but we need to take steps to maintain as many neurons as possible and to enhance their communication with one another. This means that our neurons need sufficient oxygen, glucose, nutrients and stimulation to thrive. This will include good social support and groups, physical activity, intellectual stimulation, sufficient relaxation and sleep, and, of course, a good diet.

We also need to be able to produce the correct amount of neurotransmitters (the chemical messengers) that will be able to cross the synapses and attach onto receptors in the brain cells. This is necessary because poor synaptic activity impairs brain function. Various factors can affect brain-cell health and neurotransmitter production, including inflammation (the body's response to harmful stimuli), blood-sugar imbalances, toxins, hormone imbalances, stress and insufficient key nutrients. These will be discussed in the different stages of the programme that follows.

Don't consider that forgetting things is a normal part of growing older. It is an indication that the brain is deteriorating and in the longer term it could affect your overall cognitive function and memory.

# The fear of Alzheimer's

There are an estimated 35.6 million people globally living with dementia. The numbers are expected to double every 20 years, rising to 115.4 million in 2050, mainly due to an ever-ageing population. In the US alone there will be an estimated 11–16 million individuals aged 65 and older who will be diagnosed with Alzheimer's.

The first symptoms of Alzheimer's are depression, irritability, confusion and forgetfulness. One of the problems, however, is that brain deterioration is now thought to begin decades before symptoms show.

Alzheimer's disease is a neurodegenerative disorder characterized by a decline in cognitive function. The latest research on the condition suggests that there are a number of contributing factors in the body, including oxidative stress, inflammation, mitochondrial dysfunction (causing energy imbalances) and the accumulation of certain toxic protein compounds. Underlying many of these factors are the effects of raised blood sugar and insulin – and for this reason Alzheimer's has been termed type-3 diabetes. Not only does high blood sugar promote inflammation, but also the excess insulin in the body, caused through blood-sugar imbalances, reduces the body's ability to clear out amyloid plaques – a hallmark of Alzheimer's disease.

The good news is that making the dietary and lifestyle changes outlined in this programme can reduce your risk of developing the condition.

## ALZHEIMER'S DISEASE – ARE YOU AT RISK?

The risk factors for Alzheimer's are

➤ Advancing age
➤ Family history of Alzheimer's disease
➤ Carrying the ApoE4 genetic variant
➤ Certain bacterial infections
➤ Vascular risk factors (e.g. diabetes, atherosclerosis, high blood pressure)
➤ History of head trauma
➤ High homocysteine levels
➤ Nutrient deficiencies
➤ Silent strokes (some people have strokes without ever knowing it. These so-called silent strokes either have no easy-to-recognize symptoms, or the person affected doesn't remember them. But they do cause permanent damage in the brain)
➤ Central obesity (i.e. high waist-to-hip ratio)

## Homocysteine and your risk of cognitive decline

Homocysteine is a naturally occurring amino acid produced as part of the body's methylation process (the biochemical process that occurs in the body to clear hormones, neurotransmitters and toxins). Elevated levels of homocysteine are known to be a risk factor for cardiovascular disease and have been shown to predict and correlate with the rate of cognitive decline. In addition, various research studies, including the results of the Framingham Study, published in the New England Journal of Medicine in 2016, has revealed that individuals who have high levels of homocysteine have almost double the risk of developing Alzheimer's disease compared to those with low levels.

Numerous factors, such as medications, genetic variations, smoking, alcohol, advancing age and obesity, contribute to elevated homocysteine levels. The good news is that certain B vitamins, such as folate, vitamins B12, B6, B2 (riboflavin) and betaine can help the body to maintain homocysteine levels within a healthy range. Homocysteine can be measured through a blood test by either your GP or through a home test kit. Various research studies suggest that homocysteine-lowering B vitamins can arrest cognitive decline and improve memory in people over the age of 50 with or without mild cognitive decline. Those with mild cognitive decline and raised homocysteine who were given B vitamins were shown to have a significant reduction in shrinkage of the medial temporal lobe, which is the specific area of the brain that shrinks in sufferers of Alzheimer's disease.

*The latest estimates suggest that in the US alone there will be 11–16 million individuals aged 65 and older who will be diagnosed with Alzheimer's by 2050.*

*The good news is that making the dietary and lifestyle changes outlined in this programme can reduce your risk of developing the condition.*

# How to use this book

**Whatever your age or current health concerns, this book is designed to maximize your cognitive function, performance and mood. You will also learn that you can have a brain that allows you to experience and enjoy life fully, performing to your optimal health and ability. But how do you do it?**

I suggest that you read through the first section of the book so that you understand the principles behind the diet. You will find a week-by-week explanation of each stage of the plan with background information covering the dietary and external influences that contribute to poor brain health and how to correct them.

This is followed by the practical section of the book, The Brain Boost Diet Plan on page 50, to guide you at the outset of your diet. It includes advice on fasting as an option for faster cleansing and repair, a quick-look list of what foods to avoid and what to aim to eat, plus the basics of exercise – essential for good brain health. It also contains sample menus, which focus on the four stages of the diet.

If, however, you are wondering if there is anything you can do to build better brain health now and want to get started immediately, go straight to The Brain Boost Diet Plan, read that and then dive straight into my four-week diet using the meal planner to guide you.

My suggested menus give you selected recipes for each of the four weeks of the diet, concentrating on the stages of: Cleanse, Renew, Protect and Revitalize.

Then follow recipes for optimum brain health, starting with the basics, to make your own ferments, such as sauerkraut and yogurt, if you would like to.

By following my four simple steps, you will discover a healthier body and brain for life. Remember, your brain is an organ that's connected to everything else happening in your body. Fixing your brain starts with fixing imbalances in your body. That is why many people also feel more energized, lose weight and enjoy improved overall mood as a result.

**All the recipes** are low-sugar and gluten-free, and most are dairy-free. Recipes have been given symbols for Paleo, vegetarian and vegan diets as below. But you can often make a recipe Paleo or vegan, for example, by simply substituting the dairy with the alternatives that are also listed in the ingredients.

## KEY

 **PALEO**

 **VEGETARIAN**

 **VEGAN**

# THE DIET PROGRAMME AT A GLANCE

The diet is focused on a low-carbohydrate, gluten-free, Mediterranean style of eating, but with a greater emphasis on plant-based foods, lean proteins and healthy fats. It is broken down into four weeks to make it easy to follow, but all the recipes have been carefully designed to optimize the health and function of your brain. I suggest you follow the suggested four-week meal plan, but you can simply select your favourite recipes from the book and use those to create your own meal plan if you prefer.

### WEEK ONE: CLEANSE

The first stage of the programme is a seven-day detox to cleanse the body and brain of trigger foods and toxins. This includes eliminating certain foods, sugar, additives and preservatives. The cleansing process also involves limiting continued exposure to external toxins, as well as supporting the detoxification processes of the body. This first week sets the stage, which will be followed throughout the plan, of adopting a low-sugar, low-carb and gluten-free approach to eating.

### WEEK TWO: RENEW

The focus here is on healing the body, including the gut, the blood–brain barrier and improving brain-cell function with sufficient healthy fats, protein and nutrients. Whether you are seeking to boost your mood, speed up your thinking or improve your memory, feeding your body daily with the most beneficial nutrients and foods is essential to rebuild your brain.

### WEEK THREE: PROTECT

For long-term brain health and performance, you need to flood your body with brain-protective antioxidants, increase oxygenation and lower inflammation. This stage will include key foods and nutrients to protect the brain.

### WEEK FOUR: REVITALIZE

If you struggle with low mood or memory, you might need additional nutrients to improve the balance of your neurotransmitters. In addition, for long-term improvements, making lifestyle changes is vital; whether it's dealing with stress or too little sleep, lack of exercise or insufficient mental stimulation, addressing each one of these will improve brain function and health.

# WEEK 1: CLEANSE

The first week is focused on removing the key toxins known to affect brain health and function. Research has shown that the cornerstone of all degenerative diseases, including brain disorders, is inflammation. But in our everyday life we are exposed to some of the major promoters of inflammation including sugar, refined carbohydrates, gluten and other toxins. By removing these triggers, you will immediately start to feel better and think more clearly.

At the end of Week One, you will have cleansed your body and become more accustomed to eating a diet with reduced carbohydrates and without gluten but based on fresh foods in preparation for renewal in Week Two. Here's why and how.

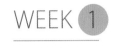

# The problem with sugar

**Blood sugar and insulin imbalances are now at epidemic proportions. Obesity and type-2 diabetes are increasing rapidly and, as we have seen, Alzheimer's is now termed type-3 diabetes because of its connection with insulin insensitivity, a key symptom of type-2 diabetes. You might have read that a diet high in carbohydrates, and particularly sugars, increases your risk of diabetes, but studies now show that such a diet also poisons your brain.**

Remember that not all carbohydrates are harmful, but the refined carbs found in processed foods such as cakes, sweets, sugary syrups, fruit juices, fizzy drinks, cookies and biscuits, pasta, breads, breakfast cereals and other processed grains will have a very different effect on your blood sugar than the slower releasing ones found in vegetables and pulses (beans, peas and lentils). Additionally, eating whole plant foods with plenty of fibre, including small amounts of beans, non-gluten whole grains, nuts and seeds, keeps toxins moving out of your body and keeps your gut bacteria healthy. A healthy gut means a healthy brain.

Although glucose is our brain's fuel source, an excess will actually impair its function. Glucose can enter our cells only through the production of insulin, which is made by the pancreas. When we eat carbohydrate foods which are frequently in the form of sugars in the modern diet, the pancreas produces insulin to push the resulting glucose into the cells. Healthy cells are very responsive to insulin, but when constantly exposed to high levels of it (caused by eating processed foods high in sugar and other carbohydrates) our cells start to desensitize their response, creating insulin resistance. This resistance leads the body to produce higher insulin levels, which causes unstable blood sugar and eventually dangerously high levels of glucose in the blood.

You don't have to be type-2 diabetic to have a problem. Insulin resistance can arise gradually after many years of unstable blood sugar levels and also from the gradual accumulation of excess weight, especially around the tummy. Even before someone is diagnosed with diabetes, having unstable blood sugar inflicts plenty of damage-promoting inflammation and glycation (the process in the body where sugar and protein molecules combine to form very harmful molecules). This affects hormones and disrupts the balance of the neurotransmitters, which not only affects how we think and feel, but also results in brain-cell damage and degeneration.

*Although glucose is our brain's fuel source, an excess will actually impair its function.*

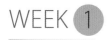
*Neurotransmitters are your main mood and brain regulators.*

Another type of damage caused by high blood-glucose levels is glycation, which occurs when glucose in the blood attaches itself to proteins, causing tissues and cells (including those in the brain) to become stiff, inflexible and dysfunctional. Our brain is very vulnerable to this type of damage, which can result in the brain tissue shrinking. You can find out whether glycation is damaging your tissues by asking your doctor for a haemoglobin A1c (HbA1c) blood test. This measures the extent to which the haemoglobin protein within your red blood cells has been glycated (damaged) by elevated blood sugar levels. Ideally, your blood-sugar level should be less than 5.7 per cent.

## How you experience low blood sugar

If you've ever experienced low blood sugar, perhaps because you haven't eaten for a while, you will be aware of how it can affect your brain. When blood sugar crashes, our brain is deprived of fuel and it stops working effectively. You might feel shaky, get a headache or blurred vision, find it difficult concentrating or feel irritable. But equally, high blood sugar is one of the major triggers of inflammation in the brain, which will cause neurons to die and speed up brain ageing. Blood sugar imbalances also influence our mood.

This is because changes in insulin levels alter the production of neurotransmitters by influencing the transport of the precursors needed for their production.

Neurotransmitters are your main mood and brain regulators. When blood sugar increases, there's a depletion of key neurotransmitters such as serotonin, epinephrine and dopamine. At the same time, certain vitamins and minerals important in their production also decline, including B vitamins and magnesium. Low levels of serotonin will result in low mood and depression, falling dopamine can also result in depression and a lack of motivation. However, by altering the balance of protein, fat and carbohydrates in your meals, you can alter the levels and balance of these neurotransmitters.

## THE LOW-CARB, LOW-SUGAR APPROACH

Reducing your overall carbohydrate intake, and in particular refined carbs and sugar, is vital for brain health.

As well as reducing sugary drinks and foods, you will need to reduce your overall carbohydrate consumption, particularly from grains, which typically make up the bulk of our carbohydrate intake. My four-week programme is a low-carbohydrate plan with a greater focus on healthy fats, protein and vegetables.

Switching to a low-carb, low-sugar diet might seem daunting at first, but after a few days on the diet you will start to notice the difference in how you think and feel. The great news is that as you switch to a low-carb diet with sufficient healthy fats and lean protein, you will put an end to cravings and mindless eating. You will enjoy feelings of fullness and satisfaction after meals without needing a pick-me-up snack.

Many people will also find that they will naturally lose weight. Being overweight and/or obese, as well as having diabetes, are major risk factors for cognitive decline, and losing weight is an additional benefit effect for many people following the diet.

In this first week, we will focus on foods that release their sugar (glucose) slowly into the bloodstream, and this will be followed throughout the four weeks of the diet plan. These types of foods are referred to as having a low glycaemic load (GL). Refined white starchy foods (breads, pasta, white rice, potato, cookies, cakes, biscuits, crackers, and so on), sweetened drinks and many fruits are high-GL foods. Meat, poultry, fish, eggs, nuts, seeds, vegetables,

*After a few days you will start to notice the difference in how you think and feel.*

beans and pulses, fats and oils have a lower GL content. Vegetables are a far superior source of carbohydrate because they do not impact on blood sugar to the extent that grains do, plus they contain important antioxidants and phytonutrients. They also have fewer calories, are easier to digest and often have more fibre.

## Which carbohydrates?

Low-carbohydrate diets mean different things to different people. The one I am promoting here is a diet that is lower in carbohydrates than standard dietary recommendations, but still includes slow-releasing carbohydrates and fibre for overall health, including gut health.

**For a healthy brain you need to avoid:**
- ➤ Added sugars, processed foods and drinks
- ➤ Gluten (wheat, barley, rye)

**The major source of carbohydrates to include in the diet will be:**
- ➤ Vegetables (including starchy vegetables such as beetroot/beet, carrot, parsnip, sweet potato)
- ➤ Some whole fruit
- ➤ Pulses (peas, beans and lentils)
- ➤ Occasional gluten-free grains (such as gluten-free oats, quinoa, brown or red rice, buckwheat, amaranth)

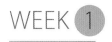

## How much carbohydrate?

The exact amount of carbohydrate you should be eating will depend on many things, including your activity levels, current health and weight. But by focusing on carbohydrates from vegetables, occasional gluten-free grains, and beans and pulses, and limiting overall fruit intake, it is unlikely to be higher than 100g/3½oz or 150g/5½oz per day (this is the amount of carbohydrate by weight and not the weight of the carbohydrate-rich food). If you are insulin resistant or diabetic, it is important to speak with your doctor or consultant before changing your diet, particularly if you are taking any medication.

To keep the carbohydrates down in the diet all you need to do is limit starchy foods to one portion (see box), once or twice a day depending on your activity levels. The best types of starchy foods to eat are beans and pulses (including lentils and chickpeas), root vegetables (such as beetroot/beet, carrot, celeriac, swede/rutabaga, turnip and sweet potato) and squash, including butternut and pumpkin, and occasional gluten-free grains (such as gluten-free oats, quinoa, and brown or red rice).

Limiting carbs minimizes insulin production and ramps up fat metabolism, so it can also be useful if you want to shift a few pounds. By including lean protein (particularly fish, eggs, beans and pulses), eating nutritious vegetables and fruits, and staying satisfied with delicious healthy-fat foods (e.g. fish, eggs, nuts and seeds), you can enjoy a wide range of foods and meals without feeling deprived.

## THE PERFECT PORTION

**To keep carbs down, one serving is:**

➤ **Fruit** 1 medium piece (such as an apple), a small handful fresh fruit salad or two small satsumas

➤ **Gluten-free grains** 60g/2¼oz/⅓ cup cooked brown rice or quinoa (or a small fist-sized portion)

➤ **Starchy vegetables** ½ medium sweet potato, or 120g/4¼oz/1 cup cubed butternut squash or pumpkin (or 1 large handful)

➤ **Pulses** (peas, beans and lentils) 80g/2¾oz/½ cup cooked pulses (or 1 small handful)

Including a variety of these lower glycaemic carbohydrates provides valuable fibre for digestive health as well as important antioxidants and nutrients for brain health.

*By including lean protein, eating nutritious vegetables, fruits and delicious high-fat foods, you can enjoy a range of meals without feeling deprived.*

## WHAT ABOUT KETOSIS FOR IMPROVING BRAIN HEALTH?

**Some programmes to support brain health recommend a ketogenic diet, to balance blood sugar, lower inflammation and aid weight loss more aggressively.**

This diet restricts carbohydrates to between 30g and 50g per day. By doing so, this enables the body to produce special fats called ketones, which the body uses as fuel in place of glucose when blood sugar is exhausted and liver glycogen is low, which occurs on a very low-carb diet. The brain can produce ketones in cells (known as astrocytes). These are very protective for the brain, and this is why a ketogenic diet appears to be effective for certain disorders, such as epilepsy and Alzheimer's disease.

Although a ketogenic approach, when planned correctly, can be effective, maintaining it can be difficult. If you suffer with hypothyroidism, for example, drastically cutting carbs can impair thyroid function, making your symptoms worse. It is often low in fibre, which can deplete the levels of beneficial gut flora, which are also essential for long-term health. So although a ketogenic diet might be beneficial in the short-term, for a longer-term approach to support brain function a low-carbohydrate, antioxidant-rich style of eating is recommended.

## How much sugar are you eating?

Sugars are found naturally in foods such as fruit, vegetables and grains, or as lactose in milk products. The main concern, however, is focused on added sugars, usually in the form of sucrose (table sugar), syrups and high-fructose corn syrup. It is estimated that a third of added sugar consumption comes from sugar-sweetened drinks, a sixth comes from foods such as chocolates, ice creams and cookies, but half comes from everyday foods such as ketchup, salad dressings and bread. New guidelines from the World Health Organization and the UK government recommend that we all aim to reduce our intake of added sugars (including the sugar present in honey, syrups and fruit juices) to 6 teaspoons a day, or 30g/1oz. To put this into context, a typical can of fizzy drink contains about 9 teaspoons of sugar.

One particular form of sugar that has received a bad press is fructose. Although fructose is naturally present in fruit, it can be harmful when processed and added to products or drinks, or used in large amounts. One of the main concerns surrounding fructose is how it is processed by the body. Fructose is almost exclusively metabolized by the liver.

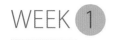
When we eat a lot of it, much of it is converted into fat. This leads to an increase in triglycerides, which increases the risk of heart disease. Excess fructose consumption has also been linked to skin ageing, diabetes, gout, cognitive decline and weight gain.

That's not to say that you should avoid whole fresh fruit – especially the lower-glycaemic fruits such as berries, avocados, cherries and citrus fruits. They are packed with antioxidants, fibre, vitamins and minerals. The fibre content helps to slow down the speed at which the sugars are digested and metabolized, avoiding sudden surges in blood sugar levels; however, you do need to watch your consumption, and I recommend that you limit consumption to no more than two portions of whole fruit a day. Fruit juice should be avoided completely – a glass of fruit juice contains about 8–12 teaspoons of sugar. When sugar is in liquid form, whether it's a soft drink or fruit juice, the fructose and glucose hit the liver faster. This means that the liver will convert much of the sugar into fat and quickly raise blood sugar and insulin, which can promote inflammation.

## SUGAR CALCULATOR

**To calculate how much sugar you are eating:**
- ➤ Look at the food label for the sugar content in the per-serving column (not per 100g/3½oz)
- ➤ Divide that number in grams by 4 to get the number of teaspoons
- ➤ If you are consuming dairy, subtract the first 4.7g/⅛oz per 100g/3½oz of sugar, as this is lactose (the natural sugar in dairy)
- ➤ Look at how much you intend to eat – it might be more than the per-serving amount

**Be label aware**
- ➤ If sugar is one of the first ingredients on the list, don't consume it
- ➤ Look out for other names for sugar, such as fruit purée, agave, coconut sugar, maple syrup, high-fructose corn syrup (HFCS), honey, palm sugar
- ➤ Look at the sugar per 100g/3½oz. Choose products that contain less than 5g per 100g/3½oz

## Do you have a problem with blood sugar?

**Keeping your blood sugar balanced is vitally important for the health of your brain. If you have any of the following common symptoms you may have poor blood-sugar control:**

- ➤ You crave sweets and carbs between meals
- ➤ You are irritable if you skip meals
- ➤ You crave coffee or sugar for energy
- ➤ You feel shaky or lightheaded
- ➤ You experience fatigue after meals
- ➤ You have difficulty losing weight
- ➤ You have abdominal fat – your waist is larger, or equal to, your hip size

## SWEETER ALTERNATIVES

Most of us like sweetness, and there are many sugar alternatives on the market, but most of them are no better for you than table sugar. You can use a small amount of fruit to sweeten certain dishes, but there are also other options you can use as natural sweeteners, although try to use them in moderation:

➤ **Xylitol and erythritol** These are sugar alcohols and are lower in calories than regular sugar. Whereas sugar contains 4 calories per gram, xylitol contains 2.4 calories and erythritol just 0.24 calories per gram. They pass through the system almost unchanged, without any of the harmful metabolic effects of excess sugar, although a high intake of xylitol can result in digestive upsets. They are available in granular form so are an easy replacement for sugar in recipes, although you might need less as they are sweeter.

➤ **Stevia** is fast becoming a popular low-calorie sweetener. It is extracted from the leaves of the plant *Stevia rebaudiana* and is incredibly sweet with virtually no calories. It also has a low GI and is very low in fructose. Stevia is available in liquid or granular form. As it is much sweeter than sugar, you will need to use much less of either type in recipes.

➤ **Monk fruit** (luo han guo) is a natural sweetener similar to stevia, but it is not as readily available. The mongrosides in the fruit appear to have antioxidant properties as well as benefits for diabetes, and they have potential anti-cancer properties. Monk fruit has no impact on blood sugar levels, with a zero GI and 30 per cent fructose. Use in a similar way to stevia in recipes.

➤ **Yacon syrup** comes from the yacon tuber from South America. The syrup tastes a little like molasses but has a low glycaemic index (GI) (between 1 and 5). This is mainly because it contains a large amount of inulin, a fructo-oligosaccharide (FOS) that tastes sweet but is not digested and acts as a prebiotic fibre, helping to feed the gut's beneficial bacteria. It contains about 40 per cent fructose, so it is best used sparingly.

➤ **Rice Malt Syrup** Rice malt syrup (sometimes labelled brown rice syrup) is made from fermented cooked rice and is a blend of complex carbohydrates, glucose and maltose. Although it has a higher glycaemic index (GI) than yacon syrup and does not offer the same prebiotic benefits, it is completely fructose-free. Use it sparingly.

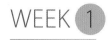

# The problem with gluten

**No single dietary protein is a more potent trigger of neurological problems than gluten. Gluten is made up of two groups of proteins: glutenins and gliadins. These proteins are poorly digested, which means gluten is able to cross the gut barrier either intact or only partially broken down. When this happens, the undigested gluten molecules alert the immune system to leap into action, because it sees them as a foreign substance to be attacked. The result is an assault on the gut lining, promoting inflammatory chemicals (known as cytokines), which affect the whole body, including the brain.**

Gluten sensitivity arises when the body produces elevated levels of antibodies against gliadins. These then promote further damage through the production of more inflammatory compounds. Antigliadin antibodies can also directly attack proteins in the brain that appear similar to the gliadin protein, resulting in yet more damage, because our own immune system has mistaken our own tissues, including our nervous tissue, for gluten. In fact, it is now well documented that gluten sensitivity is common in people suffering with neurological conditions. Remove the gluten and you can often resolve many of these symptoms. Remember, however, that you can experience neurological symptoms without having any gut or digestive symptoms at all – so don't assume that just because gluten does not cause you any gut symptoms it is OK for your body and brain.

## GLUTEN AND THE GUT

There are other ways gluten can affect the brain and body. The immune response towards gluten can leave the walls of the intestine compromised, resulting in what is known as "leaky gut" or intestinal permeability. Once you have developed leaky gut, you are more likely to experience additional food sensitivities, and the ongoing inflammatory response can also increase your risk of developing autoimmune conditions. In fact, gluten is more likely to cause auto-antibodies, because the amino-acid sequences in its structure are very similar to those of proteins in the human body, including the brain tissue. Eating gluten can therefore trigger an autoimmune attack against brain and nervous tissue. In a similar way to leaky gut, all these immune reactions to gluten can also break down the blood–brain barrier – the thin lining that protects a large part of the brain. This in turn allows a whole range of potential toxins to enter the brain and cause damage.

Coeliac disease, which is an autoimmune disease, is different from gluten sensitivity. If you have coeliac disease, when you eat gluten it sets off an autoimmune reaction that can eventually lead to complete destruction of the villi, the tiny finger-like projections lining the small intestine. These are vital for the absorption of nutrients. Therefore, as they are gradually destroyed, your body not only becomes inflamed but also malnourished. As with gluten sensitivity, you can be coeliac without having any digestive symptoms at all. In fact, many of the symptoms associated with coeliac disease involve the brain and neurological system; these include depression, cognitive impairment, dementia, epilepsy, autism, brain fog, migraines and mood disorders.

There is another way gluten can affect our brain. As gluten is broken down in our body it produces a mixture of protein molecules called polypeptides. These can cross the blood–brain barrier and bind to the brain's morphine receptors forming gluteomorphins, which create a sense of feeling high. This is the same response as that caused by opiate drugs, which suggests that gluten can also be addictive. It also explains why some reactions to gluten include a sense of brain fog, behavioural problems, cravings and mood swings. Gluten, therefore, has the ability to change our biochemistry, affecting our brain's pleasure and addiction centre – and you do not have to be coeliac to be affected.

*Some reactions to gluten include brain fog, behavioural problems, cravings and mood swings.*

## COMMON SOURCES OF GLUTEN

**The following grains contain gluten:**

| | |
|---|---|
| ➤ Barley | ➤ Rye |
| ➤ Bulgur wheat | ➤ Semolina |
| ➤ Couscous | ➤ Spelt |
| ➤ Farina | ➤ Triticale |
| ➤ Kamut | ➤ Wheat |
| ➤ Matzo | ➤ Wheat germ |
| ➤ Oats (often contaminated with gluten) | |

**Gluten is commonly found in the following products, so check labels carefully:**

| | |
|---|---|
| ➤ Beer | ➤ Malted drinks |
| ➤ Cakes, cookies, crackers, breads, pasta, and so on | ➤ Many cereal bars |
| | ➤ Many commercial soups |
| ➤ Breaded and battered foods | ➤ Marinades |
| ➤ Canned beans in sauce | ➤ Marmite |
| | ➤ Oats (unless certified gluten-free) |
| ➤ Cereals | |
| ➤ Certain cuts of meat, such as ham, sausages, salami | ➤ Pastries |
| | ➤ Quorn products |
| | ➤ Roasted and coated nuts, seeds, crisps |
| ➤ Frozen fries | ➤ Sausages |
| ➤ Gravy | ➤ Seitan |
| ➤ Instant hot drinks | ➤ Soy sauce, teriyaki sauce |
| ➤ Ketchup and other condiments | |
| ➤ Malt vinegar | ➤ Stock cubes |

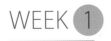

## Problem foods

For some people, going gluten-free might not be enough to manage declining brain function or inflammation. Studies have shown that proteins in other foods can cross-react with gluten. This means the proteins in certain foods are similar enough to gluten that they trigger the immune system to react. These foods include dairy, oats, yeast, millet and corn.

The most common food that cross-reacts with gluten is casein – a protein found in dairy. If you find that your symptoms are not improving on a gluten-free diet, you might wish to get tested for these cross-reactive foods, or simply avoid them altogether. In addition, if you have leaky gut, you might find that you are sensitive to other foods that may need to be avoided while you help your gut to heal (see Week Two).

Another reason why simply switching to a gluten-free diet might not be enough is that you may be consuming too many gluten-free grains. Gluten-free grains, like other carbohydrates, can lead to high blood sugar, which can promote inflammation and lead to high insulin, insulin resistance and, ultimately, type-2 diabetes.

## Paleo and vegan

All the recipes in this book are gluten-free for the reasons already mentioned. You will see that I have also highlighted whether a recipe is suitable on a Paleo, vegetarian or vegan diet. I am not necessarily advocating any specific one of

### GLUTEN FREE

**The following are gluten-free grains, pseudo grains and starches:**

| | |
|---|---|
| ➤ Amaranth | ➤ Nut and seed flours |
| ➤ Arrowroot | ➤ Potato/sweet potato |
| ➤ Banana flour | ➤ Quinoa |
| ➤ Buckwheat | ➤ Rice |
| ➤ Coconut flour | ➤ Sorghum |
| ➤ Corn | ➤ Soy |
| ➤ Gram flour | ➤ Tapioca |
| ➤ Millet | ➤ Teff |

these diets, but in essence I am advocating a combination of the three. These diets all focus on real, whole, fresh food that is sustainably produced.

A healthy Paleo diet excludes all grains, beans and pulses, and dairy products, and focuses on low-glycaemic-load (low-GL) vegetables and fruits, healthy fats and lean animal protein and seafood, which ideally is sustainably raised or grass-fed.

A healthy vegan approach (which is a vegetarian diet but excluding any animal produce, such as eggs) will include some pulses, nuts and seeds for protein and use gluten-free whole grains sparingly.

Both approaches, however, focus on eating mostly plants – lots of low-glycaemic vegetables and some fruit – and should represent 75 per cent of your diet and your plate.

# Toxins and your brain

✣ **It would be impossible to write a brain-health programme without focusing on the negative impact of environmental toxins, heavy metals and pollutants on our brain. We are not only what we eat and drink, but also what we breathe, touch and can't eliminate.**

The food, drink and medications that we consume need to be detoxified, as do all the other chemicals to which we are exposed on a daily basis. These include heavy metals, air pollution, bacteria, alcohol, cleaning chemicals and cigarette smoke, to name but a few. We are, each and every one of us, gradually accumulating hundreds of chemicals as we go through life. Our body and brain are under daily assault. Staying healthy involves a healthy liver-detoxification system, sufficient antioxidants to protect the body against toxins and a healthy gut and blood–brain barrier.

We cannot totally avoid exposure to toxins, however. Problems arise when our immune system loses tolerance to chemical exposure and begins to react to them. When this happens we can start to react to

*We are, each and every one of us, accumulating hundreds of chemicals as we go through life.*

a wide range of chemicals and metals such as perfumes, detergents, car exhaust fumes, foods and additives, and even jewellery. You might find yourself having skin reactions, asthma, headaches, brain fog, fatigue or memory problems. Often such reactions will drive inflammation in the body, which can in turn affect brain health and function.

## Nourishment to fight toxins

✣ Many organs are involved in the detoxification process; the main are the liver, gut, skin, lungs and kidneys. These organs make use of various enzymes, transporters and elimination pathways to recognize and disable toxins.

It is the liver that undertakes by far the greatest share of the work and requires a vast array of nutrients to function optimally. This is why focusing on nutrient-dense foods is so important; for example, the liver detoxification pathways need a good supply of antioxidants to help counter the damaging effects of free-radicals, plus they require amino acids, B vitamins, vitamin C, magnesium, iron and zinc, among others, to detoxify optimally.

To avoid reactions, there are several mechanisms that we need to support. For many people, glutathione, which is the body's most powerful antioxidant, is depleted. Low glutathione can also be linked to leaky gut and a compromised blood–brain barrier. Poor liver detoxification can exacerbate symptoms as can chronic inflammation in the body and a loss of immune balance, which can be linked to imbalances in beneficial gut bacteria, low vitamin D and omega-3 deficiency. There are a number of functional medicine tests that can help to determine toxic load, liver detoxification function and loss of chemical tolerance, which you can undertake in collaboration with a qualified practitioner trained in functional nutrition.

Everybody can benefit from including key nutrients and foods that support liver detoxification naturally and increase antioxidant levels. In addition, using nutrients to improve the gut barrier and blood–brain barrier, and lowering inflammation in the body and brain is also beneficial.

## Glutathione support

Glutathione is essential for protecting the brain and supporting detoxification by helping to remove toxins from the body. Although our body produces it naturally, when we are stressed, or if we eat a poor diet, drink alcohol or are exposed to other toxins, levels of glutathione become depleted. Low levels can lead to inflammation and low tolerance to chemicals.

Certain foods and nutrients help the body to recycle glutathione in the body naturally, which, together with taking supplements, can help to lower inflammation, raise levels and improve detoxification. Glutathione is also important for healing a leaky gut and the blood–brain barrier.

## NUTRIENTS AND FOODS THAT BOOST GLUTATHIONE ARE:

➤ **N-acetyl-cysteine** (NAC) (derived from cysteine-rich foods such as broccoli, chicken, cottage cheese, eggs, fish and shellfish, oats, onion, red pepper, ricotta cheese, soy beans, turkey and yogurt)

➤ **Alpha lipoic acid** (ALA) (found in beetroot/beet, broccoli, Brussels sprouts, carrot, lean red meat, liver, peas, spinach, tomato)

➤ **L-glutamine** (found in beans and legumes, cabbage, eggs, lean meat, liver, nuts, poultry, seafood)

➤ **Selenium** (selenium-rich foods include Brazil nuts, chicken, eggs, halibut, liver, sardines, spinach, turkey)

➤ **Cordyceps** (a medicinal mushroom available as a powder, see page 45)

➤ **Milk thistle** (active ingredient is silymarin) available as a supplement

➤ **Acetyl glutathione** (available as a supplement and can be boosted by whey protein powder)

# LIVER DETOX FOODS

**Our health and wellbeing is dependent on how effectively our body removes and inactivates toxins from the body. One of the main ways that the body rids itself of everyday toxins is through the liver.**

In fact, the liver is one of the hardest-working organs in the body. It works tirelessly to detoxify the blood, produce the bile needed to digest fat, break down hormones and store essential vitamins, minerals and iron. Various foods and nutrients are known to support detoxification in the liver. These include the B vitamins, vitamins C and E, magnesium, choline, iron, selenium and protein-rich foods.

**To enhance the body's natural detoxification try to include some of these key foods:**

- Artichoke
- Beetroot/beet
- Berries, cherries and pomegranate
- Choline-containing foods: asparagus, broccoli, cauliflower, eggs, fish, leafy greens, liver, mushrooms, oysters
- Citrus fruits
- Cruciferous vegetables such as broccoli, Brussels sprouts, cabbage, cauliflower, kale, rocket/arugula, watercress
- Dandelion root (available ground as a coffee replacement)
- Garlic
- Ginger
- Green tea
- Herbs, including coriander/cilantro, dill, mint, parsley, rosemary
- Onions
- Turmeric

# How to reduce your toxic exposure

Environmental chemicals and toxins are present in a vast number of everyday items. With careful choices we can reduce many of these. As part of the cleansing process you also need to start reducing your exposure to toxins in the food choices you make.

## ENVIRONMENT

➤ **Don't use pesticides** or herbicides in the garden.

➤ **Choose haircare and skincare products** without added alcohol, sodium lauryl sulfate, parabens, phthalates or other petrochemicals.

➤ **Avoid aluminium**-containing antiperspirants and antacids.

➤ **When carpeting your home**, opt for natural fibres or hardwoods, rather than standard carpets, which are usually treated with chemicals.

➤ **Think twice** before you opt for waterproof and flameproof furniture coverings and clothes.

➤ **When painting** your home or office, opt for paints labelled low- or no-VOC. Paints and finishes release low-level toxic emissions into the air for years after application.

➤ **Take steps to control the levels of dust**, bacteria and moulds in your home and office. Make use of indoor plants. Consider using an air filter and/or ionizer to reduce the particulates in the air.

➤ **Swap chemically-based household cleaners** for natural cleaners, such as spirit vinegar and bicarbonate of soda/baking soda.

➤ **Reduce your exposure** to low-level EMFs (electro-magnetic fields) by restricting your mobile phone use and removing all but the most essential electrical items from your bedroom.

➤ **If you are exercising** out of doors, stick to traffic-free zones.

➤ **Avoid passive smoking** wherever possible.

# FOOD & DRINK

➤ **Buy organic food** where possible and affordable. In particular, use organic dairy products (milk, cheese, yogurt), meat and eggs.

➤ **Wash** all fruit and vegetables before eating.

➤ **Avoid eating the larger oily fish** such as swordfish, tuna, marlin and shark. These are higher in mercury and chemical pollutants, so switch to the small oily fish such as sardines, mackerel, pilchards and anchovies.

➤ **Keep cooking temperatures low**, preferably below 200°C/400°F/Gas 6. Meat and fish that are cooked until well done or very browned (as in frying, grilling or barbecuing) can contain carcinogenic chemicals.

➤ **Reduce** your alcohol intake or avoid alcohol.

➤ **Avoid damaged fats**: trans- and hydrogenated fats in processed foods, and vegetable and seed oils (unless labelled cold-pressed) that have been heated. The healthy fats (those from oily fish, nuts, seeds and cold-pressed seed oils) help you to produce bile. This helps to excrete certain toxins from the body.

➤ **Try not to drink** bottled water from soft plastic containers; often chemicals from the plastic leach into the water. Mineral waters in glass bottles are safer, or use your own steel or hard plastic bottle, filled with filtered tap water.

➤ **Avoid food additives** such as colourings, preservatives, sweeteners and other flavour enhancers.

➤ Avoid sipping your take-away through a plastic lid.

➤ **Don't microwave plastics** – use glass or ceramic containers instead.

➤ **Make sure that any plastic** containers you use for drinking, food storage or smoothie shakers are free from bisphenol-A (BPA).

➤ **Replace any Teflon** cook- and bakeware with uncoated glass, clay, stone, enamel and stainless steel versions.

➤ **Try not to use cling film**/plastic wrap or cooking foil. Replace with paper wraps such as baking parchment.

# WEEK 2: RENEW

Now that we have ditched potentially harmful foods from the body and enhanced detoxification and cleansing, it is time to start healing the body and brain with potent healing foods and nutrients.

This week particular attention is given to restoring gut health, the addition of probiotics and prebiotics, nourishing the blood–brain barrier and improving brain-cell function with the right type of fats, amino acids, vitamins and minerals.

At the end of Week Two you will have learned about the importance of tackling any underlying digestive symptoms, restoring a healthy balance of friendly bacteria in your gut, as well as nourishing your brain and nervous system with the right fats and supportive nutrients. This will enhance the cleansing process of Week One and start to improve your cognitive function and brain performance in preparation for longer-term protection in Week Three.

# Our gut – our second brain

**As I have explained, if you're struggling with ongoing issues such as depression, anxiety, brain fog or poor memory, you need to first start looking at the health of your gut. A growing body of evidence shows that our beneficial gut bacteria support positive mood and emotional well-being. This is why our gut is sometimes dubbed our second brain.**

In our gut there is what is known as the enteric nervous system, which consists of some 100 million neurons that are embedded in the walls of the long tube of our gut, which starts at the oesophagus (the tube from our mouth to our stomach) and ends at the anus. Its nerve cells are bathed and influenced by the same neurotransmitters that affect our brain, so the gut can upset the brain just as the brain can upset the gut.

The gut also contains important bacteria. Our body is the dwelling place for about 100 trillion bacteria and other microbes, collectively known as our microbiome. They fulfil an array of important jobs, including breaking down our food, making nutrients, fighting off infection and supporting our immune system. In fact, about 80 per cent of our immune system lies within our gut, and it's our friendly microbes that help the gut's immune system to work properly. These friendly microbes

*About 80 per cent of our immune system lies within our gut.*

also help to prevent the gut lining from becoming leaky (as explained on page 20), which is essential in maintaining a healthy immune system.

In our gut lining there are special cells and antibodies that prevent foreign molecules from getting through the mucus barrier into the underlying tissues. If these invaders manage to get through because our gut is leaky, they trigger the immune cells in the underlying tissue to launch an inflammatory attack sparking inflammation, which can manifest throughout the body.

## Inflammation and its link to the gut

Research is finding that our microbiome plays an important role in our mental health and the risk of certain neurological disorders; for example, it has been demonstrated that patients with Parkinson's disease often suffer from leaky gut, and it appears that an increase in gut leakiness enhances inflammation as well as the production of a unique protein, called alpha-synuclein, both of which are characteristic of this disease. Since inflammation is the mechanism that is thought to underlie virtually every degenerative condition, it is becoming clear that the integrity of the lining of the

*It is easy for our gut bacteria to be adversely altered, whether it's through stress, environmental toxins, medications, or inappropriate food choices.*

gut, and the balance of bacteria in it, plays a fundamental role in determining the degree of inflammation in the body. One of the most important elements involved in maintaining gut-wall integrity is the balance and diversity of the microbes that live within the gut.

It is easy for our gut bacteria to be adversely altered, whether it's through stress, the overuse of antibiotics, exposure to environmental toxins, medications, and even inappropriate food choices, and this in turn can affect the integrity of the gut lining. For this reason, my diet looks beyond the brain and incorporates many foods and nutrients to promote a healthy gut flora and an intact gut lining.

## Ferments – feed the good bacteria

One of the best ways to improve the diversity and balance of our gut flora is to eat fermented foods daily. Naturally fermented foods contain a wide range of beneficial bacteria and yeasts that support a healthy gut flora. Good examples include kimchi, sauerkraut, raw pickles, kefir, kombucha, tempeh, miso, natto and raw cheese, such as some brands of Brie, Caerphilly and Cheshire, for example.

Fermented foods are incredibly nutritious. Some are outstanding sources of essential nutrients; one such example is vitamin K2, which helps to prevent arterial plaque build up and heart disease. Just 15g/½oz of natto daily can provide all the K2 you'll need. If that is not to your taste, you can also obtain some vitamin K2 in goose liver pâté and certain cheeses such as Brie and Gouda, and a little in grass-fed or organic butter. It is also found in smaller amounts in other fermented foods such as sauerkraut.

Fermented food is also a potent producer of many B vitamins essential for brain function. Fermented foods are some of the best natural foods to help remove toxins from the body (known as chelators). The beneficial bacteria in these foods are highly potent detoxifiers, capable of drawing out a wide range of toxins and heavy metals as well supporting overall health and function of the gut.

## Boost your gut with prebiotic power

To improve your gut health in the long term you need to provide the best foods for your gut bacteria. These foods are called prebiotics. Prebiotics are indigestible carbohydrates that reach the colon intact and selectively feed the many strains of beneficial bacteria there.

Prebiotics are generally classified into three different types: non-starch polysaccharides (such as inulin and fructo-oligosaccharide), soluble fibre (including psyllium husk) and resistant starch. Each of these types of prebiotics feeds different species of gut bacteria, so it is useful to include a wide range of prebiotic foods.

Our beneficial bacteria feed on prebiotic foods and produce short-chain fatty acids, which not only support colon health but also reduce inflammation in the body. In addition, prebiotic foods, but especially resistant starch, help to reduce insulin spikes and thereby lessen blood sugar imbalances, which can be so damaging for our brain.

Sources of resistant starch include: cooked pulses (peas, beans and lentils), green bananas, plantains and potato starch. Other prebiotic foods include: asparagus, chicory, dandelion greens, endive, frisée, garlic, Jerusalem artichokes, jicama, onions and radicchio. Using them raw provides the most benefits, and some of these foods are included in the recipes in this book.

## EASY WAYS TO GET MORE PREBIOTICS INTO YOUR DIET

➤ Use onions and garlic in salads, sauces, dressings, dips, soups, slow-cooked or pot meals and homemade gluten-free or Paleo crackers or breads.

➤ Add prebiotic vegetables, such as garlic, onion and asparagus to homemade fermented pickles (see Your Basic Pantry section for recipes).

➤ Look for green bananas and add them to smoothies.

➤ Shred raw Jerusalem artichokes or jicama thinly using a mandoline or grater and add to salads.

➤ Potato starch and chicory root helps to bind foods so that they can be used in baking.

➤ Try adding dandelion greens, radicchio, frisée, endive and chicory leaf to salads or add them at the end of cooking; for example, scattered over an omelette or frittata.

➤ Add a can of cooked beans or lentils to soups or stews for added fibre and protein.

➤ Add inulin flour to cookies or breads to replace some of the gluten-free flour.

# Stop being fat phobic

**For too long fat has been demonized, yet it is fundamentally important for a healthy brain. If your brain is not working well, it's time to embrace healthy fats in your diet.**

## Why do we need fat?

The human brain consists of about 60 per cent fat and is made up of primarily essential fatty acids and phospholipids. In addition, the healthy fats, particularly the essential omega-3 fatty acids and monounsaturated fats (found in avocado, olives and nuts) reduce inflammation. The essential omega-3 fats are particularly important for brain function and a healthy nervous system. They keep the neuron's membrane healthy, enabling brain cells to communicate with one another, which as we have seen, is crucial for brain function, memory, performance and mood.

Certain nutrients, such as vitamins A, D, E and K, are fat-soluble and require fat to make them available to be absorbed and utilized by the body. Deficiencies in these nutrients can have a profound effect on brain health; for example, a lack of vitamin D is associated with increased inflammation and the risk of developing conditions such as Alzheimer's, Parkinson's and depression.

Not all fats are healthy, of course. The pro-inflammatory fats include the hydrogenated or trans-fats commonly found in processed foods, ready meals and deep-fried foods. These fats make your cell membranes rigid and unresponsive, disrupting brain function and increasing degeneration. In addition, our Western diets are extremely high in omega-6 fats, which are found in many vegetable oils, including sunflower oil, corn oil and soybean oil. Our hunter-gatherer ancestors ate about as many omega-6 fats as omega-3 fats (a 1:1 ratio); today, however, the average Western diet has a ratio of between 10 and 25:1 omega-6 to omega-3 fats, which is incredibly pro-inflammatory. We are consuming far too few omega-3-rich foods and too many of these vegetable oils.

## Foods rich in omega-3

Omega-3 comes from both animal and plant sources. The primary animal sources are oily fish (anchovies, black cod, herring, kippers, mackerel, salmon, sardines and trout). The primary plant sources are chia seeds, flaxseed, hemp seeds, pumpkin seeds and walnuts.

Oily fish provides a direct source of the brain-essential fats known as eicosapentaenoic acid (EPA) and docosahexaenoic acid (DHA). Plant foods, on the other hand, provide alpha-linolenic acid (ALA), which has to be converted by the body into these active brain fats. The difficulty is that the body's ability to convert ALA is very limited, which means that if you do not eat oily fish, your levels of these protective fats is likely to be low. In addition, to support conversion it is important to keep blood sugar low and to limit omega-6 fats, as these inhibit this conversion process. Other omega-3 food sources include: leafy green vegetables, pasture-fed meat, pasture-fed eggs and non-GMO soy products.

## Are omega-3 supplements helpful?

If you have any signs of an omega-3 fatty-acid deficiency, and you avoid or eat limited oily fish, then you might benefit from a supplement. Although both EPA and DHA are important for brain health, it is DHA in particular that has the greatest benefit for brain health.

If you are looking specifically to enhance brain function, you might need a fish oil supplement higher in DHA. DHA supports the health of neuron membranes, improving the ability of neurons to release neurotransmitters, which affect how we think and feel. It also supports the growth of neuron dendrites and decreases the incidence of

neurodegenerative conditions. EPA is useful in lowering inflammation, so if you suffer with inflammatory conditions you might wish to start with a supplement that has a 1:1 ratio of EPA and DHA before switching to one with a higher DHA content. I recommend a daily intake of 1–2g high-quality fish oil.

### WATCH THE HEAT

Cooking with omega-3 oils is not recommended because heat changes the structure making them less nutritious. The most stable oils to cook with are actually saturated fats such as coconut oil. If you wish to use olive oil, only do so at low temperatures or in baking. Avoid dry-roasted nuts and seeds and opt for raw nuts and seeds. Similarly, frying oily fish at high temperatures is not recommended.

## ARE YOU DEFICIENT IN OMEGA-3 FATS?

**If you answer yes to any of the following, you should pay attention to your omega-3 levels**

➤ You never eat fish or shellfish

➤ You eat fewer than three portions of oily fish a week

➤ You struggle with chronic pain and inflammation, such as joint pain

➤ You have poor brain function; for example, you have brain fog, poor memory or poor recall

➤ You eat processed foods and/or takeaways each week

➤ You have dry skin or flaky scalp

➤ You follow a low-fat diet

➤ You suffer with hormone imbalances

➤ You suffer with depression and low mood

## What about saturated fats?

Saturated fats and cholesterol have had plenty of bad press over the decades, and yet they are important for brain health in moderation. Every cell in your body requires some saturated fats. They make up about 50 per cent of the cell membrane, and also contribute to the structure of many organs.

Cholesterol is a crucial component in the myelin sheath that coats our neurons, improving the communication between cells. It enables new synapses in the brain to grow, and provides the precursors to make phospholipids, a fatty component that is vital for brain health. It also offers protection for the brain against the harmful effects of free-radicals and is needed for the production of hormones such as oestrogen, testosterone and vitamin D, a powerful anti-inflammatory nutrient.

Deprive the brain of cholesterol and studies show that it will affect the release of neurotransmitters, which in turn affect brain function, memory and mood. Many people worry about the connection between high cholesterol and heart disease. But the truth is that there are many other factors that influence your risk of heart disease, such as high homocysteine, inflammation, glycated haemoglobin, smoking, excess alcohol consumption, lack of exercise, a diet high in carbohydrates, obesity and prolonged stress. This doesn't mean that you should be eating saturated fat in excess, however. The focus in my diet is to include more anti-inflammatory fats, primarily monounsaturated fats (such as avocado, nuts, seeds and olive oil) and essential omega-3 fats with some saturated fat from real food (present in many nuts as well as coconut oil, grass-fed lean meat and eggs) while cutting out pro-inflammatory fats, particularly vegetable oils, processed oils and hydrogenated and trans-fats.

Fats are complex, and even different types of saturated fats have different effects on the body. But is clear, of course, that the fats in a fast-food bacon cheeseburger will have an entirely different effect on your body than those in a handful of Brazil nuts.

## Coconut oil

A saturated fat, coconut oil is beneficial for brain health because it is one of the best food sources of medium-chain triglycerides (MCTs). MCTs are one of the most important superfuels for the brain, improving its function and health. Whereas our brain uses glucose for fuel once our reserves are depleted, our liver is able to use body fat as a fuel source. Ketone bodies (see page 17) are an excellent fuel for your brain and these are rapidly produced when you consume coconut oil. It is also a rich source of an important precursor molecule for beta-hydroxybutyrate, which research suggests is particularly beneficial for treating conditions such as Alzheimer's.

Another benefit of coconut oil is that it is very heat stable, making it perfect for cooking at high temperatures. For this reason it is used in some of the recipes for higher temperature cooking. It is also delicious added to drinks and desserts.

## THE BLOOD–BRAIN BARRIER

**Like the gut, we have a blood–brain barrier composed of specialist cells and blood vessels that surrounds and protects the brain.**

Of key importance is that this barrier can keep out toxins from damaging the brain cells. It is, however, vulnerable to damage – whether from blows to the head, inflammation, high cortisol from chronic stress, poor blood sugar control or ongoing exposure to environmental toxins. When the barrier becomes leaky, this can potentially result in ongoing inflammation, damage and degeneration.

The good news is that by removing the toxins outlined in Week One, balancing blood sugar, lowering stress and including key foods and nutrients, it is possible to heal the blood–brain barrier quickly.

When we have a leaky blood–brain barrier, special brain cells known as microglia cells (the brain immune soldiers) are activated, promoting ongoing inflammation and damage. Therefore it is important to lower inflammation, particularly by boosting antioxidant-rich foods in your diet.

One class of antioxidant that has a powerful anti-inflammatory effect on the brain is flavonoids: plant antioxidants found in a range of foods. These include the compounds apigenin, resveratrol, catechins, rutin and curcumin.

**Key foods to include to benefit from flavonoids are:**

- artichoke
- basil
- berries
- buckwheat

- celery
- citrus fruits
- green pepper/bell pepper

- green tea
- parsley
- red grapes
- turmeric

# WEEK 3: PROTECT

This week, the focus turns to longer-term protection and restoration of the brain cells and nervous system. There will be a greater focus on foods rich in antioxidants that will not only protect the brain cells but also improve oxygenation, lower inflammation and optimize brain function. These foods and nutrients will help you to think quicker and sharper. You will also learn how making simple lifestyle changes can also have a profound effect on how the brain ages and performs.

At the end of Week Three, you will have emphasized in your diet the foods that counter the stress on your body from previously eating foods that are lacking in nutrients and high in damaging factors such as free-radicals. You will discover the crucial role that foods rich in antioxidants and nutrients will play on the long-term functioning of your brain. And you will have built further on your dietary changes and emphases from the first two weeks of the diet in preparation for revitalizing your body and brain in Week Four.

# Tackle stress

**How stressed do you feel? Our 24/7 lifestyle means that we face significant stress all the time. In addition, one of the biggest stressors on our body is a poor, carbohydrate-rich, sugary diet that is devoid of the key nutrients our bodies require. Stress promotes inflammation, upsets brain function and destabilizes blood sugar levels. Over time, this leads to fatigue, insomnia, mood disorders, blood-sugar imbalances, inflammation, energy crashes and food cravings, among other things.**

## THE EFFECTS OF STRESS

Chronic stress can damage your brain, causing it to shrink. In addition, when we are under chronic stress, our adrenal glands produce more of our stress hormone, cortisol. This over-activates parts of our brain, depleting our body of key nutrients and disrupting our circadian rhythm (the body's natural sleep pattern, based on a 24-hour period, which coincides with the hours of darkness), which in turn affects our quality of sleep.

Stress also impacts on the production of neurotransmitters, which affect how we think and feel. This means that when we are faced with ongoing stress we are likely to have problems learning and remembering. When it comes to our health, there is one factor that is more important than almost any other and that is the health of our mind and spirit, including our attitude, social networks and a sense of connection to our community.

## Finding calm

Calming our minds and acknowledging and addressing stress is crucial for our long-term health, and yet is the one thing we tend to ignore. Learn how to relax actively – that might mean going for a walk, practising meditation, yoga or gentle exercise. Learn how to breathe deeply, and try bathing with Epsom salts to aid muscle relaxation, or treat yourself to a massage.

Of course, cleaning up your diet from mind-robbing chemicals such as caffeine, alcohol and refined sugars, as well as nourishing your body with healthy fats and nutrients, is also key to avoiding the effects of stress on the body, which I have addressed in previous weeks. There are also specific supplements that can help to support the adrenals – which are the masters behind our stress response – including magnesium, vitamin C and the B vitamins.

*One factor that is more important than almost any other is the health of our mind and spirit.*

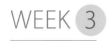

*Calming our minds and addressing stress is crucial for our long-term health, and yet is the one thing we tend to ignore.*

Spend time as well examining your beliefs, attitudes, and responses to common situations, and consider reframing your point of view or reactions to events to reduce stress.

## Nutritional ways to combat stress

As stress is so damaging for our brain, it is essential that we take steps to reduce dietary stressors, such as sugar, gluten, alcohol and processed foods to dampen the effects of stress on our long-term brain health.

Certain herbs and nutrients can help the body to adapt to ongoing stress, including ashwagandha, L-theanine, maca, rhodiola and panax ginseng, which are available in powder form, tinctures or capsules. You can also add some of the above, such as maca and medicinal mushrooms, to food, and I have included these in a few recipes in this book.

Magnesium is one of the most important anti-stress nutrients and a deficiency of it hampers adrenal function and causes anxiety. Magnesium-rich foods include figs, leafy greens, kefir, legumes, nuts and seeds, raw cacao and yogurt.

The B vitamins are also important for a healthy stress response. They are found in protein foods such as lean meat, poultry and fish as mentioned above, as well as in leafy greens, nuts, seeds and pulses.

Because the adrenal glands also hold a lot of vitamin C, if your levels are low, this is hugely stressful to the body. Aim to include vitamin C-rich sources daily, such as broccoli, peppers/bell peppers and salad leaves/greens, as well as fresh fruits, especially strawberries and citrus fruits such as oranges, lemons and grapefruit.

## IMPROVING BRAIN CIRCULATION

Your brain needs oxygen to function. Some conditions, such as low iron levels, fluctuations in blood pressure, diabetes, poor lung function and poor circulation, can also impair blood flow to the brain. An important compound called nitric oxide is produced by the body, which can improve circulation and oxygenation because it dilates the blood vessels. You can increase levels by simply exercising at a high intensity for 5–10 minutes. There are also certain foods that contain natural nitrates, and these are converted by your gut into nitric oxide.

Good foods to include to boost your circulation include beetroot/beet, cabbage, carrots, celery, garlic, lettuce, parsley, radishes, spinach, spring greens/collard greens.

The amino acids L-citrulline and L-arginine can also promote the production of nitric oxide. You can obtain citrulline in your diet by eating watermelons. L-arginine-rich foods include chickpeas, dairy, lentils, poultry, fresh pork (not processed into hams or sausages), pumpkin seeds, non-GMO soybeans and spirulina. Chillies, which contain capsaicin, as well as various plant antioxidants such as genistein, procyanidin, resveratrol, tannins and tea catechins, also increase levels of nitric oxide.

You can further boost your blood circulation with the nutrients CoQ10, ginkgo biloba, ginseng, huperzine-A and vinpocetine, plus the B vitamin, niacin. Omega-3 fats also significantly increase blood flow and nitric oxide levels (see page 38).

## Oxidative stress

Oxidation is what happens to iron when it rusts, to a sliced apple when it turns brown and to the human body when it degenerates. To protect your brain, you need to reduce oxidative damage. The process of oxidation happens as our bodies metabolize (or process) the oxygen that we breathe, and our cells produce energy from it. This process also produces free-radicals – unstable molecules that can result in damage (or stress) to our own cells, mitochondria (the energy powerhouses) and DNA.

Free-radicals are normal and necessary to some degree. Although they cause damage, they also stimulate repair. It is only when so many free-radicals are produced, and they overwhelm the repair processes, that it becomes a problem for our health, and in particular the brain cells. This is called oxidative stress. Cognitive problems arise when there is an increased free-radical attack on our brain cells.

In the case of Alzheimer's disease (see page 8), oxidative stress both facilitates some of the damage caused by amyloid-beta and prompts its formation (see also Inflammation on page 41). As brain cells (neurons) become damaged, free iron accumulates on their surfaces and within nearby cells' microglia (the brain's immune soldiers). This free iron causes more free-radical formation and drives yet further oxidative stress, and so the damage perpetuates itself.

*Oxidation is what happens to iron when it rusts, to a sliced apple when it turns brown, and to the human body when it degenerates.*

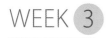

## ARE YOU GETTING RUSTY?

**Oxidative stress is a degenerative process that is destructive to all body tissues including our brain cells. There are many signs of oxidative stress – do any of the following apply to you? If you answer yes to more than six of the statements below, you need to take action to reduce your oxidative damage.**

➤ You suffer with low mood
➤ You have pigmented skin patches known as liver spots
➤ Your skin is sagging or droopy
➤ You have stretch marks
➤ You eat fewer than five portions of fruit and veg a day
➤ You eat sugary foods or white starchy foods (white bread, white rice, and so on) daily
➤ You spend a lot of time in the sun
➤ You smoke cigarettes
➤ You eat processed foods on a regular basis
➤ You eat barbecued, fried or griddled foods more than once a week
➤ You drink alcohol more than three times a week
➤ You suffer with low energy and fatigue
➤ You have memory loss and/or brain fog
➤ You have muscle and/or joint pain
➤ You have decreased eyesight
➤ You suffer with headaches/migraines
➤ You are susceptible to infections

## Aim for colour

One of the reasons a Mediterranean diet appears to be linked to a reduced risk of neurodegenerative diseases, such as Alzheimer's, Parkinson's and mild cognitive impairment, is the richness in the range of antioxidants it provides. Similarly, studies show that people who eat more plant foods have a lower risk of many age-related diseases, including high blood pressure, stroke, coronary heart disease, dementia and Alzheimer's disease, weight gain, osteoporosis and some cancers. This is probably due to the antioxidant effects of those foods, but this is not the sole reason.

These bioactive chemicals not only mop up free-radicals, preventing or slowing down the damage they cause to cells, but they also have many other benefits. Many of these compounds have the ability to "turn off" certain genes in our cells that promote inflammation, helping to prevent the blood from becoming too sticky (sticky blood is more liable to clot, causing heart attacks and strokes) and affecting blood flow in the brain. The antioxidants also keep the arteries flexible, and support the circulation and detoxification.

Vegetables, fruit, nuts, seeds, herbs and spices, for example, are rich in a range of antioxidant vitamins and minerals, including vitamins C and E, zinc and selenium, as well as a diverse range of plant compounds (called phytonutrients). As we have seen on page 35, these include polyphenols such as anthocyanidins catechins, flavonoids and resveratrol, which are now widely studied for their protective antioxidant and anti-inflammatory properties. The more colourful your plate, the greater the diversity of these plant compounds you will have in your diet.

## Inflammation

Low-grade, systemic, chronic inflammation, not apparent on the outside of the body, insidiously damages the body and brain, and is now thought to be one of the drivers of cognitive decline and mood disorders. Nutritionists often call this "inflamm-ageing" because it contributes to premature ageing.

The inflammatory process also appears to play an important role in the development of Alzheimer's disease. When high levels of amyloid-beta accumulate in the brain, they activate the body's immune response, resulting in inflammation that damages the neurons; however, including anti-inflammatory foods might help to reduce damage and the progression of the condition.

### TOP ANTI-INFLAMMATORY FOODS

➤ **OILY FISH** Anchovies, herring, mackerel, salmon, sardines and trout. Best wild-caught. (Avoid larger fish such as tuna and swordfish, as these are higher in toxins)

➤ **OMEGA-3-RICH NUTS AND SEEDS** Chia seeds, flaxseed, hemp seeds, pumpkin seeds, sesame seeds and walnuts. Include their oils and butters. Do not heat them

➤ **OTHER HEALTHY FATS** Avocado oil, olive oil, sesame oil; Brazil nuts, hazelnuts, macadamia nuts and pecan nuts

➤ **FLAVOURINGS AND SPICES** Chilli, cinnamon, garlic, ginger, nutmeg and turmeric

➤ **HERBS** (ideally fresh) Basil, boswellia, coriander/cilantro, mint, oregano, parsley, rosemary and thyme

➤ **ANTIOXIDANT-RICH FRUITS AND VEGETABLES** Especially berries, cherries, citrus fruits (including the zest), dark leafy greens such as broccoli, Brussels sprouts, kale, rocket/arugula and watercress, plus beetroot/beet, olives, onions and peppers/bell peppers. In general, the more deeply pigmented the fruit or vegetable, the greater its antioxidant power

➤ **ENZYME-RICH FOODS** Papaya, pineapple core (for example, macerated into a smoothie), sprouted seeds and sprouted beans and pulses

➤ **DRINKS** Green tea and matcha green tea powder, black tea, redbush (rooibos) tea

➤ **FERMENTED FOODS** Kefir, kombucha, miso, natto, sauerkraut, tempeh and yogurt

➤ **GREEN SUPERFOODS** Barley grass, chlorella, spirulina and wheatgrass

➤ **SEA VEGETABLES** Such as arame, kelp, kombu, nori and wakame

➤ **MUSHROOMS** Enoki, maitake, oyster and shiitake mushrooms; lion's mane and other medicinal mushroom powders

# WEEK 4: REVITALIZE

In Week Three you focused on creating a healthier environment for your brain by including high levels of antioxidant and anti-inflammatory nutrients and protecting your body against stress. Now, we will focus on revitalizing your brain through exercise and good sleep, and consuming greater amounts of the amino acids and other nutrients that are essential for brain health, mood and overall performance.

This week the focus is on balancing the production of neurotransmitters – the chemical messengers that influence how we think and feel. Through dietary changes and including certain key foods and nutrients you can boost your mood, memory and cognition. We also focus on using foods and lifestyle habits to support neurogenesis: the brain's ability to generate new neurons whatever your age.

At the end of Week Four you will experience a clearer and sharper mind. You will have a more detailed idea of the kinds of foods and nutrients that you might need for optimal performance and mood. You should also be taking time to exercise adequately and allowing yourself good sleep time for supporting overall brain function and health.

# Re-energize your brain

**It used to be thought that as we get older we are not able to grow any more neurons. Research demonstrates, however, that this is not the case. We can grow neurons as well as improving our brain circuits and connections throughout our life. Setting up good lifestyle habits now will give your body the tools it needs to keep your brain healthier for longer, whatever your age.**

Neurogenesis – the growth of new brain cells – is great news for maintaining brain health as we age, and its process is influenced by a protein called brain-derived neutrophic factor (BDNF), our brain's growth hormone. This molecule protects neurons from injury and facilitates learning and synaptic plasticity. The great news is that we can influence production of BDNF through diet and lifestyle.

## Jog your memory

We all know that exercise is good for our bodies, but did you know that it is vital for brain health too? Aerobic exercise in particular can increase BDNF, reverse memory decline and support the growth of new brain cells. In essence, exercise is like a strong fertilizer for the brain.

Exercise also supports improved communication between the cells by building new networks in the brain. This will help us to recall information and think better, and it appears that age is no barrier. It decreases stress and improves circulation and oxygenation. It also supports healthy blood-sugar levels, lowers inflammation and improves the insulin sensitivity of cells, all of which are vital for long-term brain health. In addition, regular exercise helps us to feel great by boosting levels of our feel-good chemicals.

Ideally, aim to include 30 minutes of aerobic exercise every day, such as speed-walking, running or vigorous swimming, as well as including weight-resistance work to support your muscle mass, which studies have shown can actually increase the size of specific areas of the brain and improve cognitive function. Resistance work could include using free weights, resistance machines in the gym or body-weight training such as squats, lunges and press-ups.

For brain health particularly you need to include sufficient aerobic exercise, aiming to get your heart rate up (at least by 50–60 per cent of your basal rate). You should be able to have a conversation while exercising but feel slightly breathless or break out into a sweat. If you are not used to exercise, start off slowly

*Regular exercise helps us to feel great by boosting levels of our feel-good chemicals.*

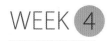
and always seek advice if you have any long-term health issues.

Prioritize your exercise slot every day: mark it in your diary and stick to it. If you need support, consider joining a gym or go to classes, enrol family members or seek support from a personal trainer. It does not have to be formal exercise sessions, of course. Aim to move regularly throughout the day. Take short breaks at work, go for a lunchtime walk, dance to music around the house or think of ways to include exercise as part of your daily commute.

## MEMORY AND LEARNING

For many people, struggling with memory lapses, and having problems recalling names or learning new skills as they age is a real concern. Such symptoms might indicate that a decline in levels of the memory neurotransmitter, acetylcholine, might be to blame. In the long term this can be linked to Alzheimer's disease and dementia. If you are concerned about memory or learning, or if you have a family history of Alzheimer's, you might wish to take supplements to boost your levels of acetylcholine. The ones you could consider are:

➤ **PHOSPHOLIPID CHOLINE:** A precursor to acetylcholine and available in capsules and granules. (A precursor is a substance from which another substance is formed.)

➤ **L-HUPERZINE** A (derived from club moss): helps to decrease the breakdown of acetylcholine, boosting levels.

➤ **L-ACETYL CARNITINE:** a structure similar to acetylcholine shown to boost cognition.

➤ **B VITAMINS** – these help in the production of acetylcholine, particularly vitamin B5 (pantothenic acid).

You do not have to take all of these, of course; often just one can make a significant difference.

**As well as supplements, choose foods rich in choline, which, as we have seen above, is a precursor to acetylcholine. These are foods naturally high in healthy fats – another reason why not to follow a low-fat diet.**

➤ Beef
➤ Cream
➤ Creamy cheeses
➤ Eggs – especially the yolks
➤ Full-fat milk
➤ Liver and organ meat
➤ Nuts
➤ Tofu

*For many people, struggling with memory lapses as they age is a real concern.*

## MAGIC MUSHROOMS

I have already mentioned numerous key foods to include for optimal brain health, but one particular group to consider for revitalizing the brain is mushrooms. Mushrooms include the culinary delights of button, chestnut, portobello and shiitake, but there are also many medicinal mushrooms that have been studied for their brain-boosting benefits. These are now readily available in powdered form or capsules to take as a supplement. The powders are delicious added to shakes and drinks or stirred into broths and soups. Here are some of the key ones that you could include.

➤ **REISHI** has been found to contain numerous anti-inflammatory and antioxidant properties, which help to protect our cells and tissues against damage from oxidative stress. Because of its strong anti-inflammatory action, it can help to relieve conditions such as arthritis, heart disease and dementia.

➤ **CORDYCEPS**, also called caterpillar fungus or tochukasu, has been demonstrated in studies to boost energy production and endurance. It is also known for nourishing the adrenal system, making it the ideal tonic to tackle stress.

➤ **CHAGA** Like all medicinal mushrooms, chaga contains complex polysaccharides known for their potent immune-supporting properties. Chaga also has an extremely high ORAC score, which is a measure of its antioxidant properties. This might be why it is regarded as an anti-ageing tonic.

➤ **LION'S MANE** The lion's mane mushroom has drawn the attention of researchers for its notable nerve-regenerative properties. About a dozen studies have been published on the neuro-regenerative properties of lion's mane mushrooms since 1991 when nerve-growth factors (NGFs) were discovered. These are key chemicals that appear to help repair the myelin (part of the neuron that transmits signals to other neurons). Some research has also shown significant improvements in people with mild cognitive impairment. It might help to improve mood and reduce depression and anxiety. In addition, lion's mane also appears to reduce amyloid-beta plaques, protein fragments that are associated with Alzheimer's.

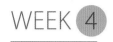

*If you struggle with feelings of depression, you might benefit from boosting your levels of serotonin.*

## MOOD BOOSTERS

Low mood and depression are common problems for many people of all ages. If you struggle with feelings of depression, loss of motivation and enthusiasm, or if you have difficulty finding joy in everyday life and hobbies, you might benefit from boosting your levels of serotonin. Low levels of serotonin are also linked to poor sleep, aggression, migraines, IBS (irritable bowel syndrome) and anxiety disorders.

Serotonin is known as the happy, feel-good neurotransmitter, which also helps us to feel calm. Its production can be influenced by oestrogen levels, which might explain why the onset of menopause can trigger low mood.

Increasing your levels of serotonin is possible naturally. Serotonin is produced from tryptophan, an essential amino acid found in protein-rich foods. Foods high in tryptophan include almonds, dairy products, legumes, meat, nuts and seeds, poultry and seafood; however, although supplements of tryptophan (and 5HTP, another precursor compound to serotonin) increase serotonin, simply adding foods containing tryptophan will not have the same effect. This is because tryptophan is directed with other amino acids into the brain by a transport system. Competition between the various amino acids for that transport system means it is more difficult to raise our tryptophan levels in the brain. One way to increase levels more effectively is to consume some carbohydrates with tryptophan-rich foods. This allows tryptophan to enter the brain more freely without competition from other amino acids, so, for example, a banana with some oats and yogurt would be a good choice.

The conversion of tryptophan to serotonin also requires certain nutrients, including iron, the B vitamins (particularly B6), niacin, methyl B12, folate and magnesium. Foods rich in B6 include bananas, beef, chicken, halibut, pistachio nuts, salmon, spinach, sunflower seeds, sweet potato and turkey. Many of these foods are also good sources of iron and L-tryptophan.

Insufficient magnesium is common in our Western diet, particularly if we exercise regularly or take certain medications such as diuretics. Certain B vitamins are also depleted when you use birth-control pills or oestrogen creams or when drinking too much alcohol. Other nutrients involved in mood include vitamin D, omega-3 fats, zinc and the amino acid, tyrosine. Again, all of these are included in the recipes to help boost your mood.

There are other ways to boost your serotonin levels. Getting outdoors and exposing yourself to bright light is an effective natural way to boost levels. Exercise has also been shown to increase serotonin levels – another reason to include exercise daily.

## Calm your mind

If you regularly feel anxious, suffer with panic attacks or find it difficult to switch off and relax, you might have an imbalance in your levels of GABA (gamma-hydroxybutyric acid – the anti-anxiety, calming neurotransmitter).

Certain supplements can be helpful to calm the body, such as L-theanine found in green tea, taurine and valerian root. Substitute your midday coffee – a stimulant that interferes with blood sugar and spikes your stress hormones – for naturally calming rooibos, chamomile or green tea, all of which have been studied for their anti-anxiety properties. Other nutrients, such as magnesium, the B vitamins, zinc and manganese, are needed for the production of GABA.

Good sources of zinc include beef, lamb, lentils, oysters, pumpkin seeds and sesame seeds (in tahini, for example). To help improve magnesium levels and to promote relaxation, try including a regular Epsom salts bath. Simply add 2 cups (480ml/17fl oz) of Epsom salts (magnesium sulfate crystals) into your warm bath and soak for 15 minutes. Your body absorbs the magnesium and sulfur through the skin, helping to calm the nervous system.

As with serotonin imbalances in blood sugar, a lack of iron also impacts on GABA production. Gluten sensitivities and toxins also interfere with GABA production. This is one reason why I include bone broth in the recipes (on page 62), which is high in glycine, an amino acid with calming properties. Foods rich in omega-3 fats (nuts, seeds, and fish such as sardines and salmon) lower inflammation and have been shown in studies to reduce anxiety.

## Get motivated

When our levels of dopamine are low, the common symptoms are: difficulty handling daily stress; an inability to motivate yourself or to start or finish tasks; and feelings of hopelessness and worthlessness. Dopamine is associated with the pleasure system in the brain, allowing us to feel enjoyment and a sense of reward, which motivates us. Insufficient levels of dopamine are most commonly linked to Parkinson's disease and addictive behaviours, such as gambling, smoking and drinking, all of which trigger the production of dopamine. Dopamine is also involved in feelings of pleasure, sexual desire and libido.

*Subsititute your midday coffee for naturally calming teas, all of which have anti-anxiety properties.*

The best foods for supporting the body's needs for dopamine are those rich in the essential amino acid phenylalanine, which are mainly found in animal products (meat, eggs, fish and cheese) as well as oats and chocolate. This means that vegans are at a greater risk of deficiency.

As with other neurotransmitters, keeping blood sugar stable, having sufficient iron, vitamin B6 and folic acid are all important for production. A lack of nutrients involved in methylation (the biochemical process that occurs in the body to clear hormones, neurotransmitters and toxins) can also play a role. These nutrients include betaine, folic acid, vitamins B6 and B12, and magnesium. A by-product of folic acid produced by healthy gut bacteria is important for dopamine production, so nourishing the gut with beneficial probiotic-rich foods and prebiotics (see Week Two) is important. If you suspect that you are low in dopamine, supplements that help to boost levels include the amino acids DL-phenylalanine and L-tyrosine, as well as vitamin B6 and the herb Mucuna pruriens. Another herb, *Bacopa monnieri*, is known for its cognitive-enhancement properties and also interacts with the production of dopamine and serotonin, improving mood.

## Tackling depression

If you struggle with feeling hopeless, sad, or otherwise mentally fragile, you are not alone. About one in three of us struggle with depression through life at some point; however, addressing depression requires a functional nutrition approach, focusing on the underlying imbalances in the body that need fixing.

A number of insufficiencies may be linked to low mood, including low B vitamins, low vitamin D, fatty acids and amino acids, gut imbalances, inflammation, low thyroid function and hormone imbalances. Additionally, tackling stress, getting sufficient exercise, sleep and being connected with family and friends are all essential. The recipes and diet plan outlined in this book are designed to address the underlying imbalances linked to the real causes of depression and low mood.

## Heal through sleep

Don't underestimate the importance of sleep. The quality and amount of sleep we get affects the health of our whole body and brain, and yet it seems that very few of us get enough.

Your total amount of sleep reduces with age at a rate of about 10 minutes per night every decade. The quality of your sleep also changes: the periods of time spent in deep sleep tend to get shorter as we age. This means that as you age, you tend to sleep more lightly and often wake up more frequently. Sleep disruptions can be related to many factors but often signal an altered circadian rhythm. This may be linked to shift working, high stress, blood-sugar imbalances or poor diet. Poor sleep also disrupts leptin and other hormones that help us to control appetite, so by improving your sleep it is likely that you can improve your food choices and weight.

# HOW TO GET RESTFUL SLEEP

➤ **ENSURE YOUR BEDROOM IS PITCH-BLACK**. Use blackout blinds if necessary.

➤ **IS YOUR BEDROOM TOO NOISY?** If so, consider whether you can install double-glazing, wear ear plugs or make other changes to reduce the noise levels.

➤ **CHECK THE TEMPERATURE** of your bedroom – too cold or too hot can interfere with sleep.

➤ **AVOID EATING LARGE MEALS** within 2–3 hours of going to bed – this can interfere with digestion and lead to bloating and pain.

➤ **TRY A LIGHT BEDTIME SNACK**. Many people find that eating a light protein-based snack about 1 hour before bed can keep their blood-sugar levels steady overnight, helping to prevent night-time waking. When blood-sugar levels plummet in the early hours, your adrenal glands will pump out the stress hormone cortisol. Cortisol will shut off your production of the sleep hormone melatonin, making it hard for you to get back to sleep. Aim to include some tryptophan-rich foods, which is a natural precursor to the sleep hormone, melatonin. Keep the snack to just a handful of nuts, a small pot of cottage cheese or a gluten-free cracker with nut butter.

➤ **AVOID ALCOHOL LATE AT NIGHT**, as it will disrupt your blood sugar, causing sleep problems.

➤ **LIMIT STIMULANTS**. Quit smoking and cut out caffeine in the afternoon and evening. They keep your level of cortisol high, which makes it difficult for the sleep hormone melatonin to rise sufficiently to help you get to sleep. Be careful with medications – some may contain caffeine. In the same way, avoid vigorous exercise within 2 hours of bedtime. But make sure to do exercise during the day.

➤ **CLEAR YOUR BEDROOM OF AS MANY ELECTRICAL APPLIANCES AS YOU CAN BEAR TO LIVE WITHOUT**. Move the TV, radio and computer to other rooms of the house. Replace your digital alarm clock with a wind-up model. If you can't remove all the electrical items, make sure you cover the digital displays to block out unwanted light.

# THE **BRAIN BOOST**
## DIET PLAN

Now that you have read about the process of the diet and the reasoning behind adopting the kind of eating I recommend, I hope that you are ready to start on the diet. As we've learned, certain types of food are beneficial for brain health whereas others are detrimental, and all the recipes in this book are tailored to support gut health as well as nourish your brain.

This diet is designed to be for life. Although it has four key phases, in essence this style of eating will improve your health and brain function in the long-term. It will help you to feel more vibrant; it will boost your mood and keep your brain sharp as you age. Making lifestyle changes can feel daunting, but I have kept the diet simple to follow to make this lifestyle easy to adopt now and for the future.

To get you started, meal plans are suggested for each week on pages 56–9.

# Getting started

**The week before you start the diet it's best to start making some simple changes. By reducing your intake of sugar and carbohydrate gradually before you start the diet, it will make it much easier to stick to the four-week programme. This is also the best time to clear out your kitchen. By ditching your house of certain foods there is less temptation and a lower chance of a lapse.**

Cutting out sugar and gluten might feel difficult at first, but within the first week you will experience clearer thinking and feel lighter and more energized. If you want to address blood-sugar imbalances, inflammation or insulin resistance aggressively, you can select the slightly lower carb dishes and/or consider intermittent fasting (see page 55).

## WHAT TO REMOVE

**ALL GLUTEN** including all baked products, breads, cereals, pasta, pastries, noodles and sauces – in fact, any products containing gluten.

**PROCESSED CARBS AND SUGARS** including gluten-free breads, pastas, sugary snacks, sweet sauces, energy bars, ice creams, fruit yogurts, jams, ketchup, soda and fizzy drinks, squash, syrups and sugar. Remember, too, that many low-fat products will also be high in sugar, so avoid them.

**INFLAMMATORY FATS** including margarines, vegetable oils, cooking oils (such as corn, grapeseed, rice bran, safflower, soy, sunflower, and so on), fried foods and takeaways.

## RESTOCK YOUR KITCHEN

By stocking your cupboards, fridge and freezer, you will save time and effort, making it much easier to stick to the programme. Use the lists below and on the following pages, and the recipes, as a guide from which you can choose a selection of ingredients that you will regularly use.

**HEALTHY FATS** include avocados and avocado oil, butter (grass-fed), coconut oil, macadamia nut oil, nuts, nut and seed butters, oily fish, olive oil, olives, seeds, cold-pressed sesame oil, and tahini. You can also purchase pure MCT oil (see page 34), which is delicious added to smoothies and hot drinks. Also include organic dairy, almond or other unsweetened nut milks, coconut milk and coconut cream, kefir and yogurt.

**HERBS, SPICES AND SEASONINGS** Keep a stash of these to add flavour and nutrition to your meals. You can buy fresh root ginger, garlic and turmeric in bulk and freeze them. To save time, you can finely grate spices or chop chillies and herbs, then freeze them in small batches.

Use a quality sea salt and enjoy low-carb condiments such as apple cider vinegar, horseradish, kimchi, miso paste, mustards, olive tapenade, pickled vegetables, sauerkraut, tamari soy sauce, tomato purée/paste and tomato salsas (I have recipes for several of these in the book).

Make use, too, of mixed spice blends, such as ras el hanout, curry blends, garam masala and za'atar. Dried sea vegetable flakes and nutritional yeast flakes provide additional nutrients and flavour, and are readily available in health-food stores. Citrus fruits, such as orange, lemon and lime, are also wonderful to add flavour to meals.

**PROTEIN** Aim to include lean protein with each meal. If you are a meat eater, select grass-fed or organic meat and eggs for a better, healthier-fat ratio. Fish and shellfish are important in the diet, and beans and pulses are included, making it ideal for vegetarians, too. The diet is very much focused on a flexitarian approach with plenty of plant-based foods with some quality meat and fish. This follows key aspects of the Mediterranean diet.

Make use of your freezer, too: buy frozen chicken breasts, fish fillets and shellfish as well as meat to keep in the freezer for standby meals.

**SUPERFOODS** These often come as nutrient-rich powders that can be a quick-and-easy way to supplement your diet with additional nutrients. They can be expensive, so to keep your food bill down, limit your choice to just a few key ones. My favourites include medicinal mushroom powders particularly Lion's mane (see page 45 for more about these), lucuma, maca, green superfood (chlorella, spirulina, wheatgrass or a blend), colostrum, acai or a berry blend, and protein powders.

**PULSES** are used in the recipes to increase plant-based protein, soluble fibre and slow-releasing carbohydrates. If you like beans and lentils, buy cans of cooked pulses in water (no sugar) or dried split red lentils, frozen edamame beans, or packets of frozen tempeh or fresh tofu.

**VEGETABLES** are an essential part of the diet. As before, make the freezer your friend. Buy bags of frozen vegetables, chopped onions, sliced peppers/bell peppers, mushrooms or mixed stir-fry veggies for quick-and-easy meals. You can also par-boil and freeze vegetables in containers if you have leftovers or an excess during certain seasons.

**GLUTEN-FREE GRAINS** Some of the recipes include gluten-free grains or pseudo-grains, such as quinoa, red rice, amaranth, buckwheat and gluten-free oats. In other recipes, lower-carbohydrate alternatives are used to replace grains to keep the carbohydrate content low. In these recipes, vegetables such as cauliflower, parsnip or celeriac are used instead.

**SWEETENERS** To avoid disrupting blood sugar I have used stevia, xylitol, erythritol, lucuma, rice malt syrup or yacon syrup in small amounts in some of the recipes.

*   **FRUIT** Whole fruit is used rather than fruit juices or dried fruit. Focus on the lower-glycaemic fruits most of the time, such as berries, cherries, citrus fruits and coconut flesh.

*   **DRINKS** Water, herbal teas and green tea are allowed on the plan. Too much caffeine will upset blood sugar, so limit regular tea or coffee to one or two cups a day with no added sugar.

Some recent research is now indicating that antioxidants, such as chlorogenic acid found in coffee, can be particularly beneficial for the brain, which is why it has been included in a few recipes. Choose a quality organic coffee if you like to include coffee in your diet.

*   **BONE BROTH** makes an ideal warming and healing drink to take through the day. The diet also includes some smoothies designed to include specific brain-healthy ingredients, which can be used as a breakfast or lunch alternative if you are following a fasting day. You can also drink the vegetable water left over when you boil or steam vegetables.

*   **AVOID ALCOHOL**, with the exception of the occasional glass of red wine (once a week) if you like.

## PREPARE AHEAD

The week before you start the diet, take the time to make up your own bone broth (page 62) and fermented foods (pages 66–69) or buy these if you don't wish to make your own. Remember, too, that you can freeze stock in small containers for up to three months, so consider making a large batch of bone broth in one go to save time.

Plan each week ahead. Look through the recipe plan provided or select your own favourite recipes for the week. Make a shopping list and stick to it. This will avoid impulse buying.

Try to be savvy so that you are not constantly cooking all week: double-batch-cook some recipes and use them, or leftovers, for lunch or breakfast the following day. You can also double-batch-cook and freeze some for using later in the plan or on busy days. Consider your daily schedule and whether you need to prepare a pack-and-go lunch or breakfast, or if you are able to cook and eat at home.

## DON'T IGNORE EXERCISE

I have mentioned how important regular exercise is for brain health in Week Four. Don't ignore the benefits for overall health and wellbeing, too.

Right at the outset of the plan, focus on taking 30 minutes of exercise every day, including aerobic exercise (such as walking or running) and some weight-resistance work a couple of times a week using free weights, resistance machines or your own body weight to build your muscle mass. You will also benefit greatly from stretching and/or yoga exercises.

Exercise improves memory, learning and concentration. Vigorous exercise has been shown to be a better antidepressant than many medications. Exercise creates brain-derived neurotrophic factor (BDNF), which is basically "miracle grow" for your brain. Exercise is also a fabulous way to reduce overall stress in your body and mind. It makes your cells and muscles more sensitive to insulin, so that you don't need as much. This is an effective way to improve blood sugar balance in conjunction with my recommended dietary changes.

## SAVVY SNACKING

There will be times you may feel hungry between meals. I don't encourage snacking, as this can cause a constant release of glucose, and with it insulin. It also requires your digestive system to be constantly active rather than allowing it to rest and thereby support digestive function.

In some cases the temptation to snack is nothing to do with hunger but boredom, or for emotional reasons. In these cases, try to distract yourself, go for a walk or have a break and change what you were doing. Alternatively, try having a glass of water or herbal tea, which might be sufficient to perk up your energy. Brushing your teeth after each meal can also help to prevent evening snacking or reaching for a sweet treat.

As the meals in the diet are filling, due to the inclusion of healthy fat and protein, it is unlikely that you will need a snack, but it's nice to know that there are some options available if you do need a snack or are particularly active.

## HEALTHY SNACKS

**There is a selection of delicious snack ideas in the book, and here are some additional healthy options as well:**

➤ A handful of raw nuts or seeds
➤ Olives and slices of cucumber
➤ Chopped raw vegetables with a little sea salt
➤ Hummus or mashed avocado with vegetable sticks
➤ Slices of cooked chicken or turkey
➤ Half an avocado with sea salt and ground black pepper
➤ Hard-boiled egg
➤ Raw crackers with nut butter
➤ A few squares (30g/1oz) dark/bittersweet chocolate
➤ Protein shake (see page 78)

# THE ROLE OF FASTING

The practice of fasting is nothing new and has been employed by every culture for centuries. It has a tremendously rejuvenating impact on our immune system, body and brain. Fasting allows the body to put more energy and focus into cellular repair and immune regulation, lowering inflammation and improving detoxification and digestion. It also improves insulin sensitivity and promotes fat burning.

There are several types of fasting. The simplest, which I recommend everyone adopts, is **time-restricted eating**: when food is eaten only within a certain period of time during the day, allowing the body to go without food for at least 12 hours. Typically, this means stopping eating at around 7pm and not eating anything again until at least 7am or 8am the following day.

**Intermittent fasting**, is sometimes referred to as the 5:2 diet, which involves fasting on fewer than 500 calories for women or 600 calories for men for two non-consecutive days a week; for example, fasting on a Monday and Thursday each week. For best results, it is recommended that on the fast day you refrain from eating breakfast and have a light lunch and an early meal, and then allow sufficient fasting hours – about 16 hours or more. This means that the following day you would not eat anything until the lunchtime, or ideally even later in the day. Fasting days should also be low in carbohydrate, similar to the rest of the diet in this book.

Alternatively, the **Fasting Mimicking Diet** (FMD) has been shown in research to promote the body's innate ability to repair itself, including positive effects on a wide range of age-related and cognitive decline risk factors, such as fasting blood glucose and inflammation. This type of fasting involves following a plant based, calorie reduced diet of around 700 calories for four or five continuous days each month then reverting back to a more Mediterranean style of eating.

Another benefit of fasting is that it can also enhance the body's natural antioxidant protection and lower inflammation in the body, which is protective in the long-term for the brain.

If you do wish to consider fasting, I have included two example fast days in the meal plan for Week One (see page 56) that would work for both of these types of fasting. To follow these fast days, skip the suggested breakfast and eat the low calorie meals for lunch, dinner and a snack.

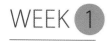
# Week 1: Cleanse

Optional fast days are marked in yellow. If you are fasting, exclude the breakfast. The lunch, dinner and optional snacks come to less than 500 calories per day.

|  | BREAKFAST | LUNCH | DINNER | OPTIONAL SNACK |
|---|---|---|---|---|
| **SUNDAY** | Sweet Greens Smoothie Bowl (p. 82) | Moroccan-Spiced Salmon Niçoise (p. 129) | One-Pot Indian Chicken (p. 144) with steamed vegetables or Cauliflower Rice (p. 167) | Coconut yogurt and berries |
| **MONDAY** | Blueberry & Walnut Granola (p. 88) with almond milk and fresh berries | Green Shakshuka (p. 99) with Breakfast Seeded Bread (p. 94) | Indonesian Fish Curry with Cauliflower Rice (p. 166) | Kale Crisps (p. 206) |
| **TUESDAY** | **FASTING DAY:** if fasting, omit breakfast **OR** Breakfast Seeded Bread (p. 94) with topping of choice | Vietnamese Prawn Salad (p. 128) | Spicy Chickpea Bowl with Turmeric Dressing (p. 115) | Brain Protein Bliss Balls (p. 202) |
| **WEDNESDAY** | Acai Berry Bowl (p. 83) | Spicy Chickpea Bowl with Turmeric Dressing (p. 115) | Soy-Braised Duck with Garlicky Leeks (p. 146) | Kale Crisps (p. 206) |
| **THURSDAY** | **FASTING DAY:** if fasting, omit breakfast **OR** Bullet-Proof Mocha Mushroom Smoothie (p. 80) | **LEFTOVER** Soy-Braised Duck with green salad | Squash & Apple Soup with Miso Butter (p. 106) with Breakfast Seeded Bread (p. 94) (omit the bread if fasting) | Brain Protein Bliss Balls (p. 202) |
| **FRIDAY** | Indian Spiced Omelette (p. 100) | Squash & Apple Soup with Miso Butter (p.106) and Breakfast Seeded Bread (p. 94) | Crispy Chicken Bites with Avocado Mayo (p. 142), sauerkraut (p. 167) and salad | Green Matcha Latte (p. 79) |
| **SATURDAY** | Blueberry & Walnut Granola (p. 88) with almond milk and fresh berries | Crispy Chicken Bites with Avocado Mayo (p. 142) and mixed salad | Garlic Broccoli, Lentil & Tomato Salad (p. 118) with Breakfast Seeded Bread (p. 94) | Green Lime Detox Shake (p. 78) |

# Week 2: Renew

|  | BREAKFAST | LUNCH | DINNER | OPTIONAL SNACK |
|---|---|---|---|---|
| **SUNDAY** | Chai-Spiced Buckwheat Crunchies (p. 84) with yogurt and berries | Jjamppong (p. 111) and Mixed Seeded Crackers (p. 211) | Thai-Spiced Burgers (p. 136) with steamed vegetables and pickles (p. 69) or sauerkraut (p. 67) | Strawberry Cream Gummies (p. 203) |
| **MONDAY** | Poached eggs with sauerkraut (p. 69) and wilted spinach | LEFTOVER Thai-Spiced Burgers with mixed salad and sauerkraut (p. 69) | Sardines with 5-Minute Romesco Sauce (p. 158) with steamed vegetables or salad | Mixed Seeded Crackers (p. 211) with nut butter (p. 74) or Smashed Lemon Chickpea Spread (p. 209) |
| **TUESDAY** | Asparagus & Salmon Mini Frittatas (p. 103) | Chicken Enchilada Soup (p. 110) | Mushroom Buddha Bowl with Miso Gravy (p. 176) | Yogurt with Fermented Apple Sauce (p. 71) or fruit |
| **WEDNESDAY** | Chai-Spiced Buckwheat Crunchies (p. 84) with yogurt and berries | LEFTOVER Mushroom Buddha Bowl with Miso Gravy | Grilled Lamb with Aubergine & Minty Chimichurri (p. 139) and vegetables | Smoky Cauliflower Bites (p. 204) |
| **THURSDAY** | Chocolate Overnight Peanut Bowl (p. 83) | Massaged-Greens Bowl (p. 116) | Quick & Spicy Mackerel Nasi Goreng (p. 164) with salad or steamed vegetables | Smoky Cauliflower Bites (p. 000) |
| **FRIDAY** | Golden Milk Turmeric Smoothie (p. 79) and scrambled eggs with wilted greens | Miso Pot Noodle (p. 117) | San Choy Bau (p. 140) with salad or steamed vegetables | Sauerkraut (p. 67) or kimchi (p. 68) and Mixed Seeded Crackers (p. 211) |
| **SATURDAY** | Chilli Breakfast Bowl (p. 101) | Speedy Nori Hand Rolls with Spicy Mayo (p. 131) and homemade pickles or kimchi (pp. 68–69) | Sticky Orange Tempeh Tacos (p. 175) and mixed salad | Superberry Swirl Kefir Ice Cream (p. 192) |

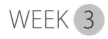
# Week 3: Protect

| | BREAKFAST | LUNCH | DINNER | OPTIONAL SNACK |
|---|---|---|---|---|
| **SUNDAY** | Savoury Waffles with Creamy Mushrooms (p. 96) | Meatball & Kale Soup (p. 108) | Hot-Smoked Salmon, Pancetta & Dill Pesto Tart (p. 151) | Pomegranate Frappuccino (p. 80) |
| **MONDAY** | Bullet-Proof Mocha Mushroom Smoothie (p. 80) | Barbecue Tempeh Bowl (p. 115) | Satay Beef Skewers with Pineapple (p. 137) | Garlic & Turmeric Chickpea Crunchies (p. 210) |
| **TUESDAY** | Golden Milk Turmeric Smoothie (p. 79) and poached eggs with spinach | Lemon & Tahini Wilted Kale & Nori Salad (p. 120) with cooked chicken breast | LEFTOVER Barbecue Tempeh Bowl | Beet Chocolate Brownies (p. 195) |
| **WEDNESDAY** | Sweet Greens Smoothie Bowl (p. 82) | Mediterranean Red Rice Salad with Pomegranate & Feta (p. 123) | Chicken Pad Thai (p. 143) | Beet Chocolate Brownies (p. 195) |
| **THURSDAY** | Indian Spiced Omelette (p. 100) | Broccoli Pizza (p. 171) with mixed salad | Salmon Tataki (p. 147) | Roasted Aubergine & Kale Tapenade (p. 208) with Mixed Seeded Crackers (p. 211) |
| **FRIDAY** | Acai Berry Bowl (p. 83) | Broccoli Tahini Cream Soup (p. 107) with Mixed Seeded Crackers (p. 211) | Cauliflower & Broccoli with Butternut "Cheese" Sauce (p. 177) | Orange Blueberry Muffins (p. 193) |
| **SATURDAY** | Orange Blueberry Muffins (p. 193) | LEFTOVER Broccoli Tahini Cream Soup with Mixed Seeded Crackers (p. 211) | Sweet Potato Gratin Fish Pie (p. 148) | Cinnamon Cream Peaches (p. 187) |

# Week 4: Revitalize

|  | BREAKFAST | LUNCH | DINNER | OPTIONAL SNACK |
|---|---|---|---|---|
| **SUNDAY** | Chocolate Raspberry Swirl Bread (p. 199) | Vegetable Ribbons with Puttanesca (p. 119) | Pan-Fried Halibut with Haricot Beans (p. 155) | Matcha Coconut Ice Cream (p. 188) |
| **MONDAY** | Breakfast Mocha No-Bake Protein Bars (p. 87) | Chicken Burrito Bowl (p. 127) | Broccoli Pizza (p. 171) with mixed salad | Green Lime Detox Shake (p. 78) |
| **TUESDAY** | Green Shakshuka (p. 99) | Vegetarian Hot & Sour Soup (p. 112) with Breakfast Seeded Bread (p. 94) or Mixed Seeded Crackers (p. 211) | Meatballs with Butternut Squash Pasta (p. 134) | Feta, Herb & Olive Muffins (p. 92) |
| **WEDNESDAY** | Feta, Herb & Olive Muffins (p. 92) | LEFTOVER Vegetarian Hot & Sour Soup with Mixed Seeded Crackers (p. 211) | Sicilian Courgetti with Olives (p. 173) | Garlic and Turmeric Chickpea Crunchies (p. 210) |
| **THURSDAY** | Poached eggs with sauerkraut (p. 67) and wilted greens | Barbecue Tempeh Bowl (p. 115) | Spiced Fish Fingers & Tartare Peas (p. 156) and Coleslaw Sauerkraut (p.67) | Cinnamon Nut Butter Cookies (p. 200) |
| **FRIDAY** | Spinach, Chickpea & Chorizo Hash (p. 89) | Vietnamese Prawn Salad (p. 128) | Quinoa Bibimbap (p. 168) | Lemon Cheesecake Layered Pots (p. 184) |
| **SATURDAY** | Caramel Apple Pancakes (p. 91) | Grilled Sea Bass with Caponata (p. 159) and mixed salad | Cauliflower Egg Fried Rice (p. 172) | Pomegranate Frappuccino (p. 80) |

# Your Basic Pantry

All the recipes in this section are healing, staple foods that will help you on your way to better brain health – and play a key part in the recipes throughout this book. Although it is sensible to stock up on ingredients for the storecupboard, refrigerator and freezer, it's also a great idea to make up a batch of key staples. This is cheaper and often healthier than shop-bought versions.

 NUTRITIONAL INFORMATION PER 100ML/3½FL OZ/SCANT ½ CUP 63 Kcals, **Protein** 3.5g, **Carbohydrates** 4.5g of which sugars 4.5g, **Fat** 3.6g of which saturates 2.3g

## Homemade Yogurt

Making your own yogurt is easy, especially if you have a yogurt maker, which are inexpensive and make preparation very quick and straightforward. Sterilize your yogurt containers before using them (see page 66). If you are sensitive to lactose, the longer you ferment your yogurt the lower the level will be. Ideally, ferment overnight or for 24 hours. Use organic milk if possible, free from hormones, antibiotics and pesticides. If you are avoiding dairy, follow the recipe for coconut yogurt instead.

Makes 1 litre/35fl oz/4⅓ cups
Preparation: 10 minutes
Cooking: 2 minutes
Fermentation: up to 24 hours

1 litre/35fl oz/4⅓ cups full-fat cow's
   milk or goat's milk
3 tbsp live natural yogurt, or
   ½ tsp probiotic powder or a
   commercial yogurt starter

**1** Heat the milk in a saucepan over a medium-high heat to just below boiling point. Remove from the heat and leave to cool until the temperature is about 38–40°C/100–104°F. This should feel warm on the skin.

**2** Add the yogurt and stir well. Transfer to a yogurt maker or pour into a clean, dry vacuum flask. Leave the milk to ferment overnight or, ideally, 24 hours. Stir well, then put in the refrigerator. It will keep for up to 1 week.

# Coconut Yogurt

NUTRITIONAL INFORMATION PER 100ML/3½FL OZ/SCANT ½ CUP 172 Kcals, **Protein** 2g, **Carbohydrates** 3.1g of which sugars 1.9g, **Fat** 16.9g of which saturates 14.6g

MAKES 800ml/28fl oz/3½ cups  PREPARATION: 10 minutes  COOKING: 4 minutes  FERMENTATION: up to 24 hours

✛ **2 x 400ml/14fl oz tins full-fat coconut milk** ✛ **1 tbsp gelatine powder or agar-agar flakes** ✛ **½ tsp probiotic powder, yogurt starter kit or 4 tbsp live yogurt if tolerated**

**1** Heat the coconut milk and gelatine in a saucepan over a medium-high heat to just below boiling point. Simmer for 2 minutes and stir well, making sure the gelatine has dissolved. Remove from the heat and leave to cool to room temperature. Stir in the probiotic powder. For a smoother consistency, put the mixture into a blender and quickly blend.

**2** Transfer to a yogurt maker or pour into a clean, dry vacuum flask. Leave the milk to ferment for 12–24 hours – the longer you leave it the more sour it will taste. After fermentation, stir well and put the yogurt in the refrigerator for 2 hours to allow the gelatine to help it set and thicken. Once firm, you can use it in recipes or on its own. Store in the refrigerator for up to 1 week.

# Cream Cheese & Whey

NUTRITIONAL INFORMATION PER 100G/3½OZ/⅔ CUP (for cream cheese) 79 Kcals, **Protein** 5.3g, **Carbohydrates** 7g of which sugars 7g, **Fat** 2.8g of which saturates 1.8g

MAKES 800ml/28fl oz/3½ cups  PREPARATION: 10 minutes, plus 24 hours straining

✛ **1kg/2lb 4oz full-fat cows or goat's yogurt**

**1** Pour the whole tub of yogurt onto the middle of a large square of muslin cloth/cheesecloth (you could alternatively use a clean pair of thin tights). Bunch the ends together around the yogurt as if you were tying it up and twist it slightly to bring the mixture into a ball inside the muslin. Secure the ends with an elastic band or string.

**2** Put the bag in a sieve/fine-mesh strainer suspended over a large glass bowl to collect the whey. Transfer to the refrigerator and leave for 24 hours. The liquid (or whey) will gradually drain out of the muslin into the bowl. Once you have collected the whey, you will be left with cream cheese inside the muslin and whey in the bowl.

**3** Put both the cream cheese and whey in the refrigerator. Store for up to 2 weeks. The whey can also be frozen. You can do this by pouring it into ice cube trays. The cubes can then be popped out for using in fermented vegetable recipes, sauces or dressings.

**P** NUTRITIONAL INFORMATION PER 100ML/3½FL OZ/SCANT ½ CUP 24 Kcals, **Protein** 3.8g, **Carbohydrates** 0.4g of which sugars 0.4g, **Fat** 0.8g of which saturates 0.2g

# Chicken Broth

A bone broth can be made from meat bones, but it is particularly easy to make using a chicken carcass. Homemade stock is very nutritious; it is rich in vitamins and minerals the body can easily assimilate. It is also ideal for soothing the digestion, healing the gut and lowering inflammation in the body, thanks to the proteins, collagen and glycine that are present in the broth. It is important to use a grass-fed or organic chicken carcass free from synthetic hormones and pesticides to avoid unnecessary toxins in the body.

Make up a large batch and freeze the stock in smaller containers to make it easy to defrost portions for using in soups and stews, for poaching meat or for making sauces and dressings. It is also delicious heated and used as a warming drink, and for my savoury smoothie recipe (Gut-Healing Savoury Blend on page 78). Adding a little vinegar is a useful way to draw out key minerals such as calcium and magnesium from the carcass. If you are roasting a chicken, remember to save all the bones to make stock afterwards.

Makes about 3 litres/105fl oz/
    12 cups
Preparation: 10 minutes
Cooking: 4–8 hours

1 whole chicken carcass, broken
    into pieces, plus the giblets and
    feet, if possible
1 whole head of garlic, cloves
    peeled (optional)
2 carrots, chopped
2 celery stalks, chopped
1 onion, quartered
1 bay leaf
1 tbsp black peppercorns
a splash of apple cider vinegar
1 strip of kombu seaweed (optional)

**1** Put all the ingredients in a large flameproof casserole or saucepan with a lid. Add 3–4 litres/105–140fl oz/12–16 cups water to cover the bones generously, then bring to the boil over a high heat. Reduce the heat to very low so that the stock is barely simmering. Cook for as long as possible – at least 3–4 hours – but you can cook for longer, about 6–8 hours. Top up with water, if needed, during cooking.

**2** Strain the stock through a sieve/fine-mesh strainer. Cool and store in the refrigerator for up to 5 days or freeze for up to 3 months. Once completely cooled, you can skim off the fat that rises to the top. (You can store the fat and use it to cook with, if you like.)

NUTRITIONAL INFORMATION PER 100ML/3½FL OZ/SCANT ½ CUP 66 Kcals, **Protein** 3.2g, **Carbohydrates** 4.6g of which sugars 4.5g, **Fat** 3.9g of which saturates 2.4g

# Kefir

The probiotic drink, kefir, is useful for improving the gut flora and is delicious used in recipes, dressings and sauces. It is made with kefir grains, which are not actually a grain but are a mother culture that digests sugar through a fermentation process. You can buy the kefir grains readily online. Although traditional milk is used, kefir can also be made with sheep's milk or goat's milk and you can make a dairy-free, vegan option using coconut or almond milk.

Kefir has many benefits, including assisting the better digestion of fats, proteins and carbohydrates. It is an ancient cultured food rich in amino acids, enzymes, calcium, magnesium, phosphorus and B vitamins. Kefir also contains several major strains of friendly bacteria: Lactobacillus caucasus, Leuconostoc, Acetobacter species, and Streptococcus species. It also contains beneficial yeasts, such as Saccharomyces, which help balance the intestinal flora, including promotion of beneficial yeast in the body by penetrating the mucosal lining.

It takes between 24 and 30 hours to ferment the cultures in milk at room temperature on colder days, but less if it is warm. Once fermented, you then store the kefir in the refrigerator and consume within 4 days.

Kefir can be used in the same way as yogurt or cream cheese. Other great uses are: in smoothies, to tenderize meat instead of yogurt, served with fruit, in a cold soup, in an ice cream recipe, in a healthy milkshake recipe, as a leavening agent, in place of buttermilk in baking, as a starter for sourdough, to make a herbed cream cheese or a fruit-flavoured cream cheese, to ferment grains or flours, to make probiotic drinks.

**Makes 1 x 1 litre/35fl oz/ 4⅓ cup jar**
**Preparation: 10 minutes**
**Fermentation: 24–48 hours**

**1 kefir starter kit or 1 sachet of milk kefir grains**
**1l/35fl oz/4⅓ cups full-fat milk or full-fat canned coconut milk**

**1** Put the kefir starter culture sachet into a sterilized 1 litre/35fl oz/ 4⅓ cup sealable glass jar (see page 66) and pour over the milk. Mix well with a wooden spoon (do not use metal, which can harm the kefir).

**2** Cover or seal loosely and leave to ferment at room temperature for 24–48 hours. Taste the mixture; it should be sour and look slightly curdled. Strain the mixture through a plastic sieve/fine-mesh strainer placed over a bowl or container. Put the kefir liquid in a clean jar in the refrigerator and reuse the grains following the recipe above. The kefir will keep in the refrigerator for 1 week.

# Beetroot Kvass

A fermented Russian beverage made out of beetroot/beets, kvass is a wonderful tonic that is traditionally served more for its medicinal effect than for its taste. Beetroot has a regenerating effect on the body, and can be used a digestive aid for those recovering from digestive ailments. Use Himalayan sea salt and avoid any salt with additives or iodine added to it, which could inhibit the growth of the beneficial bacteria. Once you have made the kvass, you can use it either as a drink on its own or blend it into a smoothie. It is particularly delicious blended with oranges and raspberries.

Makes 1 x 1 litre/35fl oz/4⅓ cup jar
Preparation: 10 minutes
Fermentation: 3 days

4 beetroots/beets, scrubbed and
   chopped into small cubes
1 lemon (optional), quartered
3–4 slices of root ginger, to taste,
   peeled
1 starter culture sachet or 5 tbsp
   whey
1 tsp Himalayan sea salt

**1** Put the beetroots/beets into a sterilized 1 litre/35fl oz/4⅓ cup sealable glass jar (see page 66) or several small jars. Squeeze the lemon quarters, if using, a little over the beetroots, then add them, followed by the ginger, starter culture and salt. Add water to fill the container, leaving a 3cm/1¼in space at the top of the jar.

**2** Make sure the beetroot is submerged in the liquid or put a weight on top to let the juice rise over the beetroot while it ferments. Cover or seal loosely. Leave the jar at room temperature for at least 2–3 days until the liquid is slightly fizzy. Strain out the beets and transfer the kvass to the refrigerator. You can drink it right away, but it's often best after a few days. As a fermented beverage, this kvass will last for at least 1 month.

**3** Save the beets for a second batch. Save about 125ml/4fl oz/½ cup of the kvass in your jar as a starter, then fill it with water again, and leave it again for a few days. Your kvass will last for at least a month in the fridge. Either discard the beetroot or eat it after the second batch.

P  V  VE    NUTRITIONAL INFORMATION PER 100ML/3½FL OZ/SCANT ½ CUP 13 Kcals, **Protein** 0g, **Carbohydrates** 3g of which sugars 1g, **Fat** 0g of which saturates 0g

# Homemade Kombucha

Known as the "immortal health elixir" by the ancient Chinese, kombucha is made from sweetened tea that's been fermented by a symbiotic colony of bacteria and yeast (known as SCOBY). It is rich in many of the enzymes your body produces for digestion, and it aids cleansing and supports liver health. As it is naturally high in sugars, even when fermented, it is best drunk only occasionally and in small amounts. In view of the sugar content, limit it to 150ml/5fl oz/scant ⅔ cup a day.

Makes 1 x 1 litre/35fl oz/
    4⅓ cup jar
Preparation: 10 minutes,
    plus 1 hour cooling
Fermentation: 3–14 days

3 or 4 black or green tea bags,
    to taste
90g/3¼oz/½ cup sugar or coconut
    sugar
1 packet of kombucha starter
    culture (SCOBY)

**1** Put the tea bags in a 1 litre/35fl oz/4⅓ cup sterilized glass jar (see page 66) and add the sugar. Pour over 600ml/21fl oz/scant 2½ cups boiling water. Stir well with a plastic spoon, then allow the mixture to cool for 1 hour or until it reaches room temperature.

**2** Add the SCOBY. Cover the container with a cloth or muslin cloth/cheesecloth and leave in a warm place for 3–7 days to brew. The liquid will become a little cloudier when ready. After 3–4 days, taste the brew. If it tastes fruity and not tea-like, it's ready, if not, leave it for a few more days and try again.

**3** Strain the mixture, but leave a little of the tea in the container with the SCOBY so that you can repeat the process to make another batch. You can keep the ready-made brew in the refrigerator for up to 4 days – it will get fizzier the longer you leave it, but it is still fine to drink.

## VARIATIONS

➤ BERRY & VANILLA  Add 1 vanilla pod/bean and a few berries to fermented kombucha. Leave at room temperature for 2–3 days.

➤ LEMON TURMERIC TONIC  Add 1 lemon, sliced, to fermented kombucha followed by a 2cm/¾in piece of peeled turmeric root and 2–3 slices of peeled root ginger. Leave to stand at room temperature for 2–3 days.

➤ CHAI SPICE  Add 2 star anise, 2 cinnamon sticks, 1cm/½in piece of peeled root ginger and 4 cloves to fermented kombucha. Leave to stand at room temperature for 2–3 days.

# Fermented Vegetables

Not only are fermented vegetables so simple and cheap to make, but by making your own you ensure that they are packed with the beneficial bacteria that is so beneficial for the gut, and so the brain. Unlike pickling, which is commonly used in many shop-bought versions (using vinegar and sugar), lacto fermenting uses salt and sometimes whey to encourage the growth of the vegetables' natural beneficial bacteria. Lactobacillus bacteria coat the vegetables, encouraging the formation of lactic acid, which supports the digestion. Fermentation also helps the B vitamins, vitamin C and, in some foods, vitamin K and minerals to become more bioavailable, and lowers the overall sugar content. Many people find ferments curb food cravings and improve the digestion. You can ferment almost any vegetable and experiment with flavours, but it is important to follow a few tips:

## FERMENTNG TIPS

➤ **STERILIZE JARS.** Place your sealable glass jars on a hot rinse cycle in the dishwasher, or put the clean jars in a warm (not hot) oven for 30 minutes.

➤ **USE ORGANIC**, fresh vegetables. Wash and dry them thoroughly.

➤ **SUBMERGE YOUR FERMENTS.** Your vegetables need to be fully submerged in the liquid – this will prevent harmful bacteria or mould from developing. You can do this by putting a few large rolled-up cabbage leaves on top, then a ramekin or a small jar on that, or use a weight if you have traditional weighing scales.

➤ **ADD SUFFICIENT SALT.** I have included measurements in the recipes below, but essentially the ratio is 1 tablespoon sea salt for 500ml/17fl oz/2 cups water.

➤ **USE QUALITY SEA SALT.** I like to use Himalayan pink salt.

➤ **TASTE THE LIQUID** after 2–3 days of fermentation – it should taste slightly sour, or even a little fizzy if it has fermented sufficiently. If not, leave it for a further few days and then retest.

➤ **CONTROL THE TEMPERATURE.** It is important to keep the temperature around 16–22°C/60–71°F. Too cold and nothing will happen, but too hot and you will destroy the beneficial bacteria. When it is warmer, the vegetables will ferment more quickly, so tasting is important.

➤ **DON'T FASTEN THE LID TOO TIGHTLY.** In warm conditions there is a slight risk that the lid could blow off, so keep the lid loose.

# Coleslaw Sauerkraut

  **V** **VE** NUTRITIONAL INFORMATION PER 100G/3½OZ/⅔ CUP 22 Kcals, **Protein** 0.7g, **Carbohydrates** 3.2g of which sugars 3g, **Fat** 0.3g of which saturates 0g

MAKES 1 x 1 litre/35fl oz/4⅓ cups jar   PREPARATION: 15 minutes, plus 15 minutes soaking and overnight softening   FERMENTATION: 3–4 days fermenting

÷1 handful sea vegetables (optional) ÷½ small white cabbage, shredded (about 400g/14oz) ÷½ red cabbage, shredded (about 400g/14oz) ÷3 carrots, shredded ÷2 shallots, finely chopped ÷2.5cm/1in piece of root ginger, peeled and grated ÷3 garlic cloves, chopped ÷1 tbsp caraway seeds ÷1 tbsp fennel seeds ÷3 tbsp sea salt

**1** If using sea vegetables, soak them in water for 15 minutes, then drain in a colander and chop. Put the cabbage, carrots, shallots, sea vegetables, ginger, garlic and seeds in a large bowl and toss together.
**2** Put the salt in a separate small bowl and add 125ml/4fl oz/½ cup warm water, then stir to dissolve. Pour over the vegetables and massage the mixture with your hands. Leave to one side at room temperature to soften overnight.
**3** Spoon the mixture into a sterilized 1 litre/35fl oz/ 4⅓ cup sealable glass jar (see page 66) or several small jars, pressing down as you go. Fill the jar with water so that the juices come to the top of the cabbage mixture. Make sure that there is a little room, about 3cm/1¼in, at the top of the jar. Put a weight on top to let the juice rise over the vegetables while it ferments. Cover or seal loosely.
**4** Leave the jar in a warm place for 7 days or a little longer if it is cooler until slightly sour. Store in the refrigerator for up to 3 months.

# Pineapple & Turmeric Sauerkraut

   **P** **V** **VE** NUTRITIONAL INFORMATION PER 100G/3½OZ/⅔ CUP 21 Kcals, **Protein** 0.6g, **Carbohydrates** 3.7g of which sugars 3.5g, **Fat** 0.2g of which saturates 0g

MAKES 1 x 1 litre/35fl oz/4⅓ cup jar   PREPARATION: 20 minutes, plus 1 week fermenting

÷½ white cabbage, shredded (about 450g/1lb) ÷¼ pineapple including the core, peeled (about 200g/7oz) ÷1 onion, finely chopped ÷1cm/½in piece of root ginger, peeled and grated ÷1 tbsp ground turmeric or 2cm/¾in piece of turmeric root, peeled and grated ÷1 tbsp fennel seeds ÷1 tbsp sea salt

**1** Put the cabbage in a large glass bowl. Chop the pineapple into small chunks and add it to the bowl with the onion. Add the ginger, turmeric, fennel seeds and sea salt. Massage the cabbage mixture with your hands for 5 minutes or until it starts to break down and become soft. Pour over 600ml/ 21fl oz/scant 2½ cups warm water and mix well.
**2** Pack the mixture into a sterilized 1 litre/35fl oz/ 4⅓ cup sealable glass jar (see page 66) making sure there is sufficient liquid covering the cabbage. If needed, put a small weight on the top, leaving about a 2.5cm/1in gap from the top. Cover or seal loosely.
**3** Leave the jar in a warm place for up to 1 week until it tastes slightly sour and a little fizzy. It will store in the refrigerator for at least 1 month.

# Beetroot Apple Kraut

   NUTRITIONAL INFORMATION PER 100G/3½OZ/⅔ CUP 26 Kcals, **Protein** 0.8g, **Carbohydrates** 4.4g of which sugars 4.2g, **Fat** 0.3g of which saturates 0g

MAKES 1 x 1 litre/35fl oz/4⅓ cup jar  PREPARATION: 15 minutes  FERMENTATION: 1 week

✛1 small red cabbage (about 600g/1lb 5oz), shredded ✛300g/10½oz beetroot/beets, grated ✛300g/10½oz apples, cored and grated ✛1 tbsp juniper berries ✛1 tbsp coriander seeds ✛2 tbsp sea salt ✛125–150ml/ 4–5fl oz/½–⅔ cup water or use a mixture of water and whey

**1** Put the vegetables and apples in a large bowl. Grind up the berries and seeds using a mortar and pestle, then put in the bowl. Dissolve the salt in the water and pour it over the vegetables. Massage the mixture, then cover it and leave it overnight at room temperature.
**2** Spoon the mixture into a sterilized 1 litre/ 35fl oz/4⅓ cup sealable glass jar (see page 66) or several small jars, pressing down as you go. Fill

the jar with enough water so that the juices come to the top of the cabbage mixture. Make sure there is a little room, about 3cm/1¼in, at the top of the jar. Put a weight on top to let the juice rise over the vegetables while it ferments. Cover or seal loosely.
**3** Leave the jar in a warm place for at least 1 week until fermented to taste – it should taste slightly sour. Transfer to the refrigerator and use within 3 months.

# Fruity Spiced Kimchi

  NUTRITIONAL INFORMATION PER 100G/3½OZ/⅔ CUP 17 Kcals, **Protein** 0.6g, **Carbohydrates** 2.9g of which sugars 2.8g, **Fat** 0.1g of which saturates 0g

MAKES 1 x 1 litre/35fl oz/4⅓ cup jar  PREPARATION: 30 minutes, plus resting  FERMENTATION: 5 days

✛1 Chinese cabbage, shredded ✛3 tbsp Himalayan pink salt ✛300ml/10½fl oz/scant 1⅓ cups warm water ✛1 small daikon, grated ✛1 carrot, grated ✛4cm/1½in piece of turmeric root, peeled and grated ✛1 tbsp smoked dried chilli/hot pepper flakes or chipotle flakes ✛2cm/¾in piece of root ginger, peeled and finely grated ✛3 garlic cloves, crushed ✛½ red onion ✛1 ripe pear, cored ✛2 tsp fish sauce (optional)

**1** Put the cabbage leaves in a large bowl. Dissolve 1 tbsp of the salt in the water, then pour it over the cabbage. Massage the leaves gently in the salt solution, then leave to soak for 1 hour. Drain and return it to the bowl. Add the daikon and carrot.
**2** Put the remaining salt into a blender or food processor and add the turmeric, dried chilli/hot pepper flakes, ginger, garlic, red onion and pear, then add 2 tbsp water and the fish sauce, if using, and

whiz to form a thick paste, adding a further 1 tbsp water if needed. Pour the paste over the vegetables and mix thoroughly. Leave to rest for 30 minutes.
**3** Spoon the mixture into a sterilized 1 litre/35fl oz/ 4⅓ cup sealable glass jar (see page 66) or several small jars and add water to cover the vegetables. Put a weight on top to let the juice cover the vegetables.
**4** Leave in a warm place for 4–5 days, or longer if it is cold. Store in the refrigerator for up to 3 months.

# Turmeric-Spiced Leftover Pickles

   NUTRITIONAL INFORMATION PER 100G/3½OZ/⅔ CUP 16 Kcals, **Protein** 1.1g, **Carbohydrates** 1.7g of which sugars 1.3g, **Fat** 0.3g of which saturates 0.1g

MAKES 1 x 1 litre/35fl oz/4⅓ cup jar   PREPARATION: 15 minutes   FERMENTATION: 2–5 days

✛½ tsp ground turmeric or 2cm/¾in piece of turmeric root, peeled and grated ✛1 tsp black peppercorns ✛1 tsp fennel seeds ✛1 tsp coriander seeds ✛½ small cauliflower, cut into florets ✛1 courgette/zucchini, cut into thick slices ✛½ red pepper/bell pepper, deseeded and cut into large chunks ✛100g/3½oz green beans, cut in half if long ✛1 tbsp Himalayan sea salt ✛2 tbsp whey (optional)

**1** Put the spices in a sterilized 1 litre/35fl oz/4⅓ cup sealable glass jar (see page 66). Arrange the vegetables in different layers in the jar. Mix the salt in 500ml/17fl oz/2 cups warm water and stir well to dissolve the salt. Add the whey to this mixture, if using.
**2** Pour over the vegetables leaving a 3cm/1¼in space at the top of the jar. Put a weight on top to let the juice rise over the vegetables while it ferments. Cover or seal loosely.
**3** Leave the jar in a warm place for 2–3 days or for about 5 days if it is cold. Store in the refrigerator for up to 3 months.

# Cucumber Dill Pickles

   NUTRITIONAL INFORMATION PER 100G/3½OZ/⅔ CUP 15 Kcals, **Protein** 1g, **Carbohydrates** 1.1g of which sugars 1.1g, **Fat** 0.6g of which saturates 0g

MAKES 1 x 1 litre/35fl oz/4⅓ cup jar   PREPARATION: 15 minutes   FERMENTATION: 3–4 days

✛1 tbsp Himalayan pink salt ✛2 tbsp whey (optional) ✛1 handful of fresh dill leaves ✛3 garlic cloves, sliced ✛1 tsp mustard seeds ✛1 tsp black peppercorns ✛1 tsp dill seeds ✛4–5 baby cucumbers, to fill a jar, or 1 cucumber cut into large chunks

**1** Dissolve the salt in 500ml/17fl oz/2 cups warm water and add the whey, if using. Stir well to dissolve the salt.
**2** Put the dill into a sterilized 1 litre/35fl oz/4⅓ cup sealable glass jar (see page 66) and add the garlic and spices.
**3** Pack in the cucumbers, leaving a 3cm/1¼in space at the top of the jar. Pour over the brine, retaining the 3cm/1¼in space at the top of the jar. Put a weight on top to let the juice rise over the cucumber while it ferments. Cover and seal loosely.
**4** Leave to ferment in a warm place for 3–4 days or for about 5 days if it is colder. Store in the refrigerator for up to 3 months.

# Blender Mayonnaise

 **V** NUTRITIONAL INFORMATION PER 1 TBSP 106 Kcals, **Protein** 0.4g, **Carbohydrates** 0g of which sugars 0g, **Fat** 11.5g of which saturates 1.8g

MAKES about 200g/7oz/¾ cup   PREPARATION: 5 minutes

✛ **2 egg yolks** ✛ **1–2 tbsp lemon juice** ✛ **½ tsp Dijon mustard** ✛ **150ml/5fl oz/⅔ cup extra virgin olive oil, omega blend oil or macadamia nut oil, or use 50ml/1¾fl oz/scant ¼ cup MCT oil or a combination of melted coconut oil plus 100ml/3½fl oz/scant ½ cup olive oil** ✛ **1 tbsp whey (optional)** ✛ **sea salt and ground black pepper**

**1** Put the egg yolks into a blender beaker. Add the lemon juice, mustard and oil.

**2** Insert the hand-held/immersion blender into the beaker and switch on. After 30 seconds the mayonnaise should start to thicken. Continue for a further 1 minute or until the mayonnaise has thickened to your liking. Season with a little salt and pepper.

**3** Stir in the whey, if using. Store in the refrigerator for up to 3 days.

# Ketchup

   **P V VE** NUTRITIONAL INFORMATION PER 1 TBSP 17 Kcals, **Protein** 0.2g, **Carbohydrates** 0.8g of which sugars 0.5g, **Fat** 1.4g of which saturates 0.2 g

MAKES about 500g/1lb 2oz/1¾ cups   PREPARATION: 15 minutes   COOKING: 20 minutes

✛ **100g/3½oz sun-dried tomatoes in oil, drained** ✛ **400g/14oz can chopped tomatoes or passata** ✛ **¼ red onion, finely chopped** ✛ **2 tbsp apple cider vinegar** ✛ **½ tsp ground cinnamon** ✛ **½ tsp smoked paprika** ✛ **½ tsp ground allspice** ✛ **1 tbsp xylitol or erythritol** ✛ **sea salt and ground black pepper**

**1** Put all the ingredients in a saucepan and bring to the boil, stirring well to dissolve the xylitol. Reduce the heat and simmer, uncovered, for 20 minutes or until the sauce is quite thick. Stir occasionally to prevent the mixture sticking to the bottom of the pan.

**2** Leave to cool, then whiz in a blender or food processor. Cool and store in a glass container in the refrigerator for up to 3 weeks or freeze for up to 3 months.

# Fruity Barbecue Sauce

NUTRITIONAL INFORMATION PER 1 TBSP 7 Kcals, **Protein** 0.2g, **Carbohydrates** 1.1g of which sugars 0.9g, **Fat** 0.2g of which saturates 0g

MAKES around 800ml/28fl oz/3½ cups   PREPARATION: 15 minutes   COOKING: 20 minutes

✢1 tbsp olive oil  ✢1 onion, chopped  ✢2 garlic cloves, crushed  ✢1 apple, cored and chopped  ✢140g/5oz can tomato purée/paste  ✢400g/14oz can chopped tomatoes  ✢4 tbsp balsamic vinegar  ✢4 tbsp apple cider vinegar ✢1 tsp Dijon mustard  ✢1 tbsp lemon juice  ✢1 tbsp xylitol or erythritol  ✢2 tbsp tamari soy sauce ✢5mm/¼in piece of root ginger, peeled and chopped  ✢½ tsp ground cinnamon  ✢1 tsp smoked paprika

**1** Put the oil in a saucepan over a medium heat and cook the onion, garlic and apple for 5 minutes to soften. Add all the remaining ingredients. Bring to the boil, then reduce the heat and simmer gently for 15 minutes or until the apple is soft and the mixture has thickened.

**2** Transfer to a blender or food processor and whiz until smooth. The sauce can be served warm or at room temperature. Store in the refrigerator for up to 5 days.

# Fermented Apple Sauce

NUTRITIONAL INFORMATION PER 100G/3½OZ/⅔ CUP 47 Kcals, **Protein** 0.5g, **Carbohydrates** 9.8g of which sugars 9.5g, **Fat** 0.4g of which saturates 0.1g

MAKES about 400g/14oz/1½ cups  PREPARATION: 15 minutes, plus making the kombucha  FERMENTATION: 24 hours

✢5 eating apples, peeled, cored and sliced  ✢½ tsp ground cinnamon  ✢4 tbsp Homemade Kombucha (page 65)

**1** Put the apples in a blender or food processor with the cinnamon. Add the kombucha and whiz until you reach your desired consistency – you might wish to retain a little texture.

**2** Spoon the mixture into a sterilized glass jar (see page 66) and cover loosely. Leave at room temperature for 24 hours to ferment, then transfer to the refrigerator. Store for up to 1 month.

# Whipped Coconut Cream

This is delicious topped on hot drinks and smoothies or used as a cake frosting or an alternative to yogurt with fruit as a treat. It's important to use full-fat canned coconut milk rather than a light version. For cakes you could flavour this with vanilla or citrus.

**Makes 125g/4½oz/½ cup**
**Preparation: 10 minutes**

400ml/14fl oz can full-fat coconut
  milk
½–1 tsp granulated stevia or 1 tbsp
  yacon syrup, to taste

**1** Put the unopened can of coconut milk upright in the refrigerator overnight – this allows the thick cream to harden at the top of the can.

**2** Open the can and scoop out the thick cream, and put it in a glass bowl – depending on the brand you will probably have about 125g/4½oz/½ cup. (The liquid underneath can be used as a drink added to smoothies or curries. You can also freeze this liquid if you don't wish to use it immediately.)

**3** Scatter the stevia over the thick cream in the bowl. Using a hand-held/immersion blender, briefly whiz until smooth and creamy (or transfer to a jug blender or food processor and whiz). Store in the refrigerator until required.

NUTRITIONAL INFORMATION PER 1 TBSP 34 Kcals, **Protein** 0.9g,
**Carbohydrates** 3.4g of which sugars 0.4g, **Fat** 1.4g of which saturates 0.1g

# Berry Chia Jam

Enjoy this delicious alternative to regular jam, which is ideal for spreading on bread or crackers (page 211), stirred into yogurt or used for adding to desserts.

Makes 150g/5½oz/scant ½ cup
Preparation: 5 minutes
Cooking: 3 minutes

130g/4¾oz/1 cup fresh or frozen
    mixed berries
1 tbsp xylitol or erythritol
3 tbsp whole chia seeds

**1** Put all the ingredients in a saucepan over a medium-low heat. If using fresh berries, add 2 tablespoons water and heat gently for 1 minute to dissolve the xylitol. (If using frozen berries, you are unlikely to need additional liquid.)

**2** Increase the heat to medium and cook gently for 2 minutes or until the mixture begins to thicken, stirring frequently.

**3** Using a hand-held/immersion blender, whiz the mixture to form a thick purée. Allow the mixture to cool – it will thicken a little more as it chills. Store in an airtight container in the refrigerator for up to 1 week or freeze for up to 3 months.

# Nutritious Nut Butters

Although nut butters are now widely available, it is also easy to make your own. You do need a good-quality food processor fitted with an S-blade or a high-speed blender to achieve a lovely smooth texture, however. I find the process a lot faster if you warm the nuts in an oven first. Put them in an oven preheated to 110°C/225°F/Gas ½ for 10–15 minutes until they are just warm. This helps their oils release faster in the food processor.

   NUTRITIONAL INFORMATION PER 1 TBSP (almond nut butter) 101 Kcals, **Protein** 2g, **Carbohydrates** 3g of which sugars 0g, **Fat** 9g of which saturates 1g

## Homemade Nut Butter

You can soak the nuts in advance and dry them out in the oven, if you like, which can make them easier to digest. For a richer flavour, lightly toast the nuts before grinding. As an approximation, the amount of nut butter created is roughly half the volume of the nuts you start with.

Makes 180g/6¼oz/1½ cups
Preparation: 5–10 minutes

375g/13oz/3 cups nuts – you can
    use a mixture or just one type,
    such as almonds, cashew nuts,
    macadamia nuts, walnuts
oil, ghee or coconut oil (optional)
herbs or spices, to taste (optional)
sea salt and ground black pepper

**1** Put the nuts in a high-speed blender or food processor and whiz until the mixture is smooth and creamy. You might need to stop occasionally and scrape down the sides with a spatula. Store in an airtight container in the refrigerator for 1–2 weeks or freeze for up to 3 months.

## VARIATIONS

➤ **WHITE CHOCOLATE MACADAMIA BUTTER**
✛50g/1¾oz/¼ cup raw cacao butter
✛1–2 tbsp xylitol or erythritol ✛250g/9oz/
2 cups macadamia nuts ✛115g/4oz/1⅓ cups
desiccated/dried shredded coconut
✛1 tsp vanilla extract ✛a pinch of sea salt

Put the raw cacao butter in a saucepan
over a medium heat and add the xylitol.
Melt gently together, then leave to one
side. Put the nuts into a high-speed
blender or food processor, add the
coconut, and whiz until the mixture starts
to become smooth. Add the vanilla extract,
the cacao butter and a pinch of sea salt,
and whiz until creamy.

➤ **SUGAR-FREE STRAWBERRY BUTTER**
✛250g/9oz/3⅓ cups desiccated/dried
shredded coconut ✛160g/5¾oz/1 cup fresh or
defrosted frozen strawberries ✛a pinch of sea
salt ✛1 tbsp xylitol or erythritol

Put the coconut into a high-speed
blender or food processor and whiz until
completely smooth. Add the strawberries,
sea salt and xylitol. Whiz until smooth
and creamy.

➤ **CHOCOLATE NUT SPREAD**
✛375g/13oz/3 cups hazelnuts ✛1 tbsp vanilla
extract ✛2 tbsp coconut, MCT or extra virgin
olive oil ✛a pinch of sea salt ✛50g/1¾oz/
½ cup raw cacao powder ✛200ml/7 fl oz/scant
1 cup water, full-fat coconut milk or coconut
kefir (optional) ✛1 tbsp granulated stevia, or
1–2 tbsp erythritol or rice malt syrup

Preheat the oven to 180°C/350°F/Gas Mark 4.
Put the hazelnuts on a baking sheet and
toast in the oven for 6–8 minutes until
golden. Put the nuts in a tea towel and rub
off most of the skins (to prevent a bitter
taste). Put the nuts in a high-speed blender
or food processor and add the vanilla
extract, oil, sea salt and cacao powder.
While blending, gradually add up to
200ml/7fl oz/scant 1 cup water, coconut
milk or coconut kefir to create a thick
paste. Sweeten to taste with stevia.

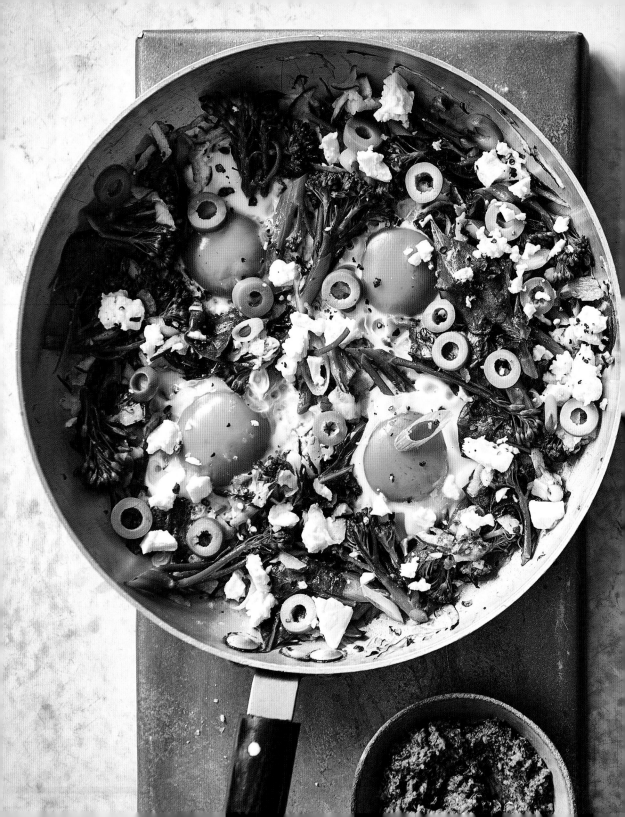

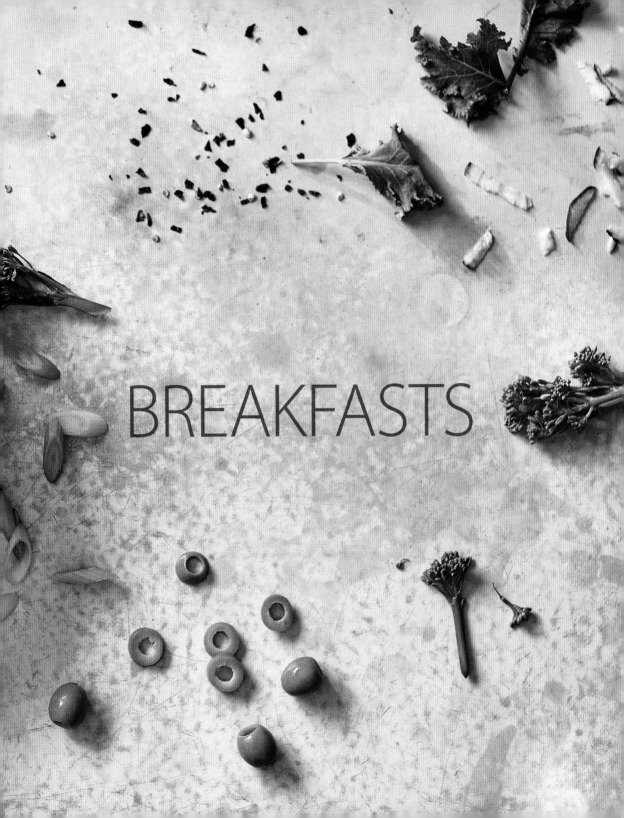

BREAKFASTS

# Green Lime Detox Shake

   NUTRITIONAL INFORMATION PER SERVING 83 Kcals, **Protein** 2.1g, **Carbohydrates** 5.7g of which sugars 0.9g, **Fat** 5.4g of which saturates 1g

SERVES 2  PREPARATION: 5 minutes

✛ 240ml/9fl oz/1 cup coconut water ✛ ⅓ cucumber, chopped ✛ zest and juice of 2 limes ✛ ½ ripe avocado, pitted and skinned ✛ 1 handful of parsley leaves ✛ 2–3 mint leaves, to taste ✛ 1 handful of spinach leaves ✛ 1 tsp supergreen powder or matcha powder ✛ 1 tsp granulated stevia, or to taste ✛ 1 handful of ice cubes

**1** Put all the ingredients into a high-speed blender or food processor and whiz until smooth and creamy. Serve immediately.

**Brain Benefits**

This smoothie is perfect for supporting detoxification pathways. Coconut water provides valuable electrolytes to hydrate the brain quickly, making this a useful pick-me-up when you feel fatigued.

# Gut-Healing Savoury Blend

 NUTRITIONAL INFORMATION PER SERVING 47 Kcals, **Protein** 7g, **Carbohydrates** 2.2g of which sugars 1.4g, **Fat** 0.7g of which saturates 0.3g

SERVES 2  PREPARATION: 5 minutes, plus making the stock  COOKING: 2 minutes

✛ 1 handful of frozen peas ✛ 1 handful of chopped kale leaves ✛ ½ courgette/zucchini, chopped ✛ 500ml/17fl oz/2 cups homemade Chicken Broth (page 62) or other meat stock ✛ a pinch of sea salt ✛ ¼ tsp ground turmeric ✛ ¼ garlic clove ✛ 1 tbsp lemon juice ✛ ground black pepper

**1** Put all the ingredients into a blender or food processor and whiz until smooth. Pour into a saucepan and warm through. Pour into mugs to serve.

**Brain Benefits**

Chicken broth is an excellent source of collagen, which is good for gut healing and lowering inflammation. The peas supply B vitamins and folate, good for production of neurotransmitters, plus carotenoids and the antioxidants catechin and epicatechin to protect the brain from free-radical damage. The smoothie is a perfect light lunch if you are following intermittent fasting days.

# Golden Milk Turmeric Smoothie

   NUTRITIONAL INFORMATION PER SERVING 77 Kcals, **Protein** 0.8g, **Carbohydrates** 13.3g of which sugars 9.3g, **Fat** 2.2g of which saturates 1.7g

SERVES 2   PREPARATION: 5 minutes   COOKING: 5 minutes

✢ **400ml/14fl oz/1¾ cups full-fat coconut milk** ✢ **½ tsp ground turmeric or 5mm/¼in piece of root turmeric, peeled and grated** ✢ **½ tsp ground cinnamon** ✢ **a pinch of ground black pepper** ✢ **1 tbsp xylitol or erythritol, or to taste** ✢ **a slice of peeled root ginger** ✢ **1 tsp coconut oil**

**1** Pour the milk into a blender or food processor and add the turmeric, cinnamon, pepper and xylitol, then whiz until smooth.

**2** Pour the mixture into a saucepan and add the ginger and oil. Simmer for 5 minutes to allow the flavour to develop. Strain and serve warm.

**Brain Benefits**

Curcumin, one of the active compounds in turmeric, is capable of crossing the blood–brain barrier, which is one reason why it holds promise as a neuro-protective agent. Known for its anti-inflammatory and antioxidant properties, it might help in the prevention and recovery of brain function in neurodegenerative diseases such as Alzheimer's.

# Green Matcha Latte

   NUTRITIONAL INFORMATION PER SERVING 45 Kcals, **Protein** 3.2g, **Carbohydrates** 0.5g of which sugars 0.2g, **Fat** 2.9g of which saturates 0.2g

SERVES 1   PREPARATION: 5 minutes   COOKING: 2 minutes

✢ **240ml/9fl oz/1 cup almond milk or coconut milk** ✢ **½ tsp matcha tea powder** ✢ **stevia, rice malt syrup or yacon syrup, to taste** ✢ **Whipped Coconut Cream to serve (optional) (page 72)** ✢ **dusting of cinnamon to top (optional)**

**1** Put the milk and matcha powder in a jug and whisk together. Pour the mixture into a saucepan, add the stevia and warm it through over a medium heat.

**2** Using a hand-held milk frother, or small whisk, froth it until hot, thick and creamy. Pour the smoothie into a mug and serve with some coconut whipped cream and a dusting of cinnamon, if you like.

**Brain Benefits**

The epigallocatechin-3-gallate (EGCG) in green tea is a powerful antioxidant known to protect brain health. Green tea also contains L-theanine, an amino acid which increases levels of neurotransmitters (the brain's messenger chemicals) known as gamma-aminobutyric acid (GABA), serotonin, dopamine (see pages 46–47), and alpha-wave activity – and might also reduce mental and physical stress.

# Bullet-Proof Mocha Mushroom Smoothie

   NUTRITIONAL INFORMATION PER SERVING 177 Kcals, **Protein** 16.1g, **Carbohydrates** 9.4g of which sugars 0.4g, **Fat** 7.8g of which saturates 2.4g

SERVES 2 PREPARATION: 5 minutes

✛ 30g/1oz/scant ¼ cup chocolate protein powder ✛ 1 tbsp raw cacao powder ✛ ½ tsp ground cinnamon ✛ 1 tbsp almond nut butter ✛ 2 tsp xylitol, erythritol or stevia, or to taste ✛ 2 tsp lion's mane mushroom powder or medicinal mushroom powder ✛ 150ml/5fl oz/⅔ cup hot or cold brewed organic coffee, yerba mate or green tea ✛ 150ml/5fl oz/⅔ cup almond milk ✛ 1 tsp coconut oil or MCT oil, melted

**1** Put all the ingredients into a blender or food processor and whiz until smooth and creamy. Serve immediately.

**Brain Benefits**

Lion's mane (see page 45) is particularly beneficial for brain health. Studies suggest it can improve cognitive function, nerve regeneration, remyelination (the repair of the covering of the nerve fibres), and increased nerve growth factor (NGF), making it useful for preventing, and even reversing, mild cognitive decline, including early Alzheimer's.

# Pomegranate Frappuccino

   NUTRITIONAL INFORMATION PER SERVING 37 Kcals, **Protein** 0.4g, **Carbohydrates** 6g of which sugars 5.6g, **Fat** 1.2g of which saturates 0.1g

SERVES 2 PREPARATION: 5 minutes, plus making the coconut cream

✛ 1 large handful of ice cubes ✛ 125ml/4fl oz/½ cup almond milk, Kefir or Coconut Kefir (page 63) ✛ 100ml/3½fl oz/ scant ½ cup pure pomegranate juice ✛ 1 tsp acai berry powder or berry powder ✛ Whipped Coconut Cream (page 72)

**1** Put all the ingredients, except the coconut cream, into a blender or food processor and whiz until smooth and creamy.

**2** Pour into glasses, then top with the whipped coconut cream and serve.

**Brain Benefits**

Pomegranate is well known for its antioxidant protective properties, which, together with the acai berry powder, makes this smoothie perfect for protecting and rejuvenating the brain.

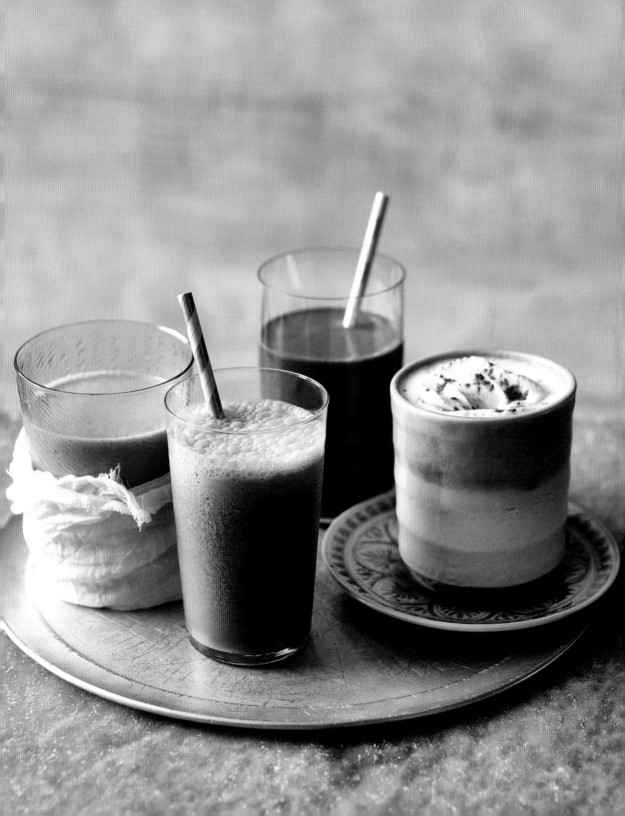

# Super Smoothie Bowls

Incredibly simple to make and more substantial than just a drink, smoothie bowls are also an easy and tasty way to eat plenty of vegetables, protein, fibre and antioxidants to help you feel fuller throughout the morning. You can also sprinkle the bowls with homemade Buckwheat Crunchies or Granola (see pages 84 and 88). To make your bowls more nutritious, aim to keep the fruit content down while increasing the protein and healthy fats. This will help to keep your blood sugar level more balanced throughout the day. There are so many different variations you can try. Here are a few examples, but have fun experimenting with your favourite ingredients. Serve in bowls with toppings of your choice.

*Smoothie bowls are an easy and tasty way to eat plenty of vegetables, protein, fibre and antioxidants.*

## Sweet Greens

NUTRITIONAL INFORMATION PER SERVING 311 Kcals, **Protein** 18.6g, **Carbohydrates** 20g of which sugars 11.6g, **Fat** 14.8g of which saturates 2.8g

SERVES 2 PREPARATION: 5 minutes, plus making the Buckwheat Crunchies

✢ 70g/2½oz kale or spinach leaves, chopped  ✢ 350ml/12fl oz/1½ cups almond milk or kefir  ✢ 30g/1oz/scant ¼ cup vanilla protein powder  ✢ 1 tsp spirulina powder  ✢ 2 tbsp chia seeds  ✢ 1 ripe pear, cored and chopped ✢ ½ small avocado, pitted, skinned and chopped ✢ a small handful of ice cubes
FOR THE TOPPING  ✢ 1 kiwi, sliced  ✢ 1 tsp chia seeds ✢ 1 tbsp unsweetened coconut flakes
✢ Buckwheat Crunchies or Granola (pages 84 and 88)

**1** Put all the smoothie ingredients in a high-speed blender or food processor. Leave to stand for 5 minutes, then blend until creamy and smooth. Top and serve.

### Brain Benefits
Spirulina is a cleanser and detoxifier that contains the mood-booster, L-tryptophan, an amino acid the body uses to synthesize serotonin and melatonin. For a probiotic boost, use kefir instead of almond milk and leave for 5 minutes before blending to allow it to thicken.

# Acai Berry Bowl

   NUTRITIONAL INFORMATION PER SERVING 206 Kcals, **Protein** 7.8g, **Carbohydrates** 21.8g of which sugars 19.3g, **Fat** 9.2g of which saturates 2.5g

SERVES 2 PREPARATION: 5 minutes, plus making the kefir

✢ **1 banana** ✢ **250ml/9fl oz/1 cup Coconut or Milk Kefir (page 63)** ✢ **1 tbsp acai or other berry superfood powder**
✢ **100g/3½oz/¾ cup frozen berries** ✢ **1 tbsp cashew nut butter** ✢ **toppings of your choice, to serve**

**1** Chop the banana and put it into a freezer bag. Exclude all the air, then seal and freeze overnight or until solid.
**2** Put all the ingredients in a high-speed blender or food processor and whiz until creamy and smooth. Top and serve.

**Brain Benefits**
A healthy gut is essential for your mental health, as imbalances in your gut flora can have a detrimental impact on your brain health, leading to issues such as anxiety and depression. Aim to include at least one serving of probiotic-rich foods such as kefir or yogurt in your daily diet. Use a berry superfood or acai powder to optimize the protective properties of this smoothie.

# Chocolate Overnight Peanut Bowl

  NUTRITIONAL INFORMATION PER SERVING 382 Kcals, **Protein** 22.1g, **Carbohydrates** 47.5g of which sugars 1.9g, **Fat** 9.9g of which saturates 1.9g

SERVES 2 PREPARATION: 5 minutes, plus overnight soaking

✢ **1 banana** ✢ **30g/1oz/scant ¼ cup vanilla or chocolate protein powder** ✢ **2 tbsp raw cacao powder**
✢ **2 tsp smooth peanut butter** ✢ **350ml/12fl oz/1½ cups almond milk or coconut milk**
✢ **80g/2¾oz/scant 1 cup gluten-free oats or buckwheat groats** ✢ **toppings of your choice, to serve**

**1** Chop the banana and put it into a freezer bag. Exclude all the air, then seal and freeze overnight or until solid.
**2** Put all the ingredients except the oats in a high-speed blender or food processor and whiz until creamy and smooth. Stir in the oats, then put in the refrigerator overnight to thicken. When ready to eat, spoon into bowls, scatter over your toppings and serve.

**Brain Benefits**
Studies have shown that chocolate affects your emotions and mood by raising serotonin levels, which might explain why people often crave chocolate when their mood is low. It also contains the compound theobromine, a mild stimulant that might also help to lift your mood.

P V VE NUTRITIONAL INFORMATION PER SERVING 269 Kcals, **Protein** 4.3g, **Carbohydrates** 32.1g of which sugars 1.3g, **Fat** 12.8g of which saturates 9.2g

# Chai-Spiced Buckwheat Crunchies

This wonderful cereal alternative is also delicious as a healthy snack and is low in sugar. Soaking the buckwheat starts the sprouting process, which makes it much easier to digest. The addition of tahini is a perfect way to add a rich creaminess to the texture.

Serves 6
Preparation: 15 minutes,
    plus overnight soaking
Cooking: 20–30 minutes

3 bags of chai tea
200g/7oz/1¼ cups buckwheat
    groats, rinsed
1 tsp ground cardamom
1 tsp ground cinnamon
a pinch of ground ginger
30g/1oz/⅓ cup raw cacao powder
2 tbsp yacon syrup or rice malt
    syrup
60g/2¼oz/heaping ¼ cup coconut
    oil, melted
1 tbsp tahini
1 tbsp lucuma powder (optional)

**1** Make up the chai tea with 300ml/10½fl oz/1¼ cups boiling water and the tea bags.

**2** Put the buckwheat groats in a large bowl. Cover with the tea, adding more water if needed to ensure that it is fully covered. Leave to soak overnight.

**3** Rinse the groats well and allow them to drain in a sieve/fine-mesh strainer. Preheat the oven to 180°C/350°F/Gas 4 and line two baking sheets with baking parchment.

**4** Put the groats in a large bowl and stir in the remaining ingredients. Mix thoroughly to make sure all the buckwheat is fully coated. Spread the mixture thinly onto the prepared baking sheets. Bake for 20–30 minutes until crisp, stirring occasionally so that the mixture does not burn. Leave to cool, then store in an airtight container for up to 4 weeks.

**Brain Benefits**

A staple in both Mediterranean and Middle Eastern cuisines, tahini is a paste made from sesame seeds. The seeds are rich in lignans, a type of plant compound known as polyphenol, and they are known to help support cardiovascular health and the circulation, and to lower inflammation.

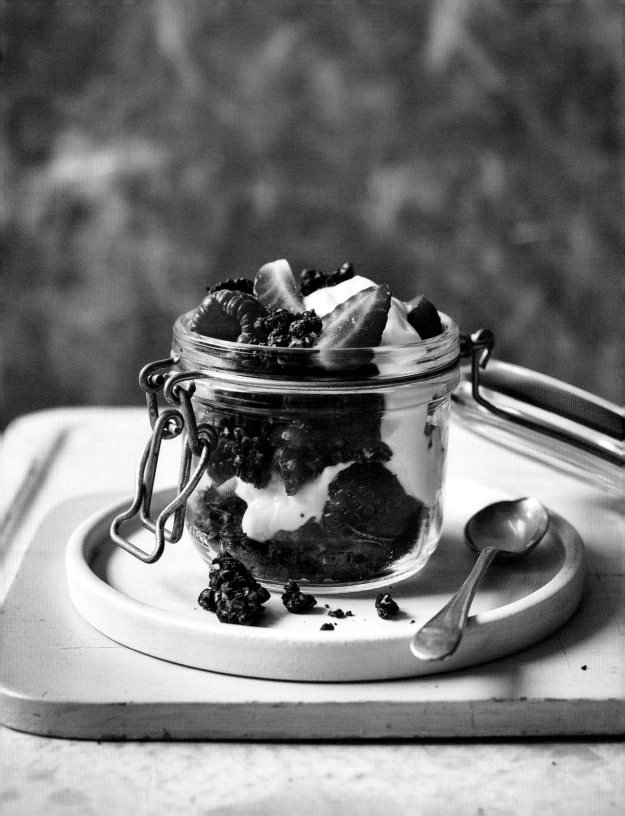

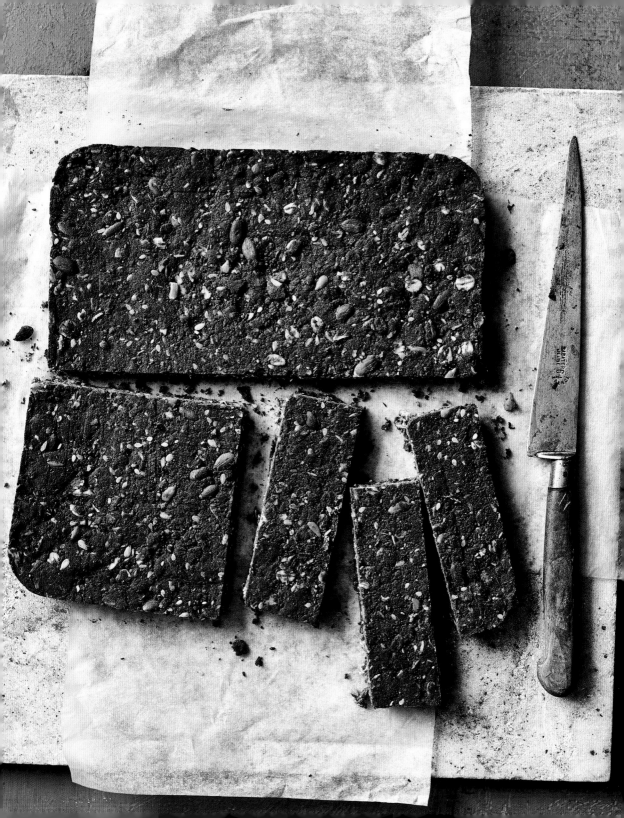

V VE NUTRITIONAL INFORMATION PER BAR 178 Kcals, **Protein** 9.3g, **Carbohydrates** 11.6g of which sugars 0.2g, **Fat** 10g of which saturates 5.1g

# Breakfast Mocha No-Bake Protein Bars

Many traditional bars are full of sugars – whether in the form of added syrups or dried fruit. My bars are much lower in carbohydrate and higher in protein, thanks to the addition of vanilla protein powder. I have sweetened them with ground xylitol. You can store them in the freezer and take them out in the morning if you want to eat a bar after a workout or later in the day.

Makes 12 bars
Preparation: 15 minutes
Cooking: 2 minutes, plus 1 hour
    freezing

60g/2¼oz/heaping ½ cup coconut
    oil
1 heaping tbsp almond nut butter
2 tbsp xylitol or erythritol, finely
    ground
100g/3½oz/1 cup gluten-free oats
90g/3¼oz/¾ cup vanilla protein
    powder
30g/1oz/⅓ cup raw cacao powder
1 tsp espresso ground coffee
1 tbsp vanilla extract
3–4 tbsp almond milk
4 tbsp mixed seeds
1 tbsp chia seeds

**1** Line a 20cm/8in square baking pan with baking parchment. Put the oil, nut butter and xylitol in a saucepan over a medium-low heat and melt gently for 1–2 minutes until the oil has melted and the xylitol has dissolved.

**2** Put the oats in a food processor or mixing bowl and add the protein powder, cacao powder, espresso coffee and vanilla. Pulse or stir to briefly mix. Add the oil mixture and stir to combine. Add enough almond milk to form a stiff, soft dough. Stir in the seeds and beat well to form a sticky dough.

**3** Spoon the mixture into the prepared pan, then spread out and smooth the surface. Put in the freezer for 1 hour to harden. Cut into 12 bars and store in the refrigerator for up to 1 week or freeze for up to 3 months.

## Brain Benefits

Despite its bad press, coffee in moderate amounts can be healthy as it contains hundreds of biologically active compounds, including caffeine, chlorogenic acid, trigonelline, cafestol and kahweol. Various studies suggest that it might help to boost brain function, and reduce the risk of Alzheimer's disease and Parkinson's disease.

# Blueberry & Walnut Granola

A delicious pink granola, this breakfast favourite has the addition of puréed berries. It contains a wealth of omega-3 nuts and seeds to nourish the brain and to provide plenty of protein to keep the body energized. It is delicious served with milk, kefir or a milk alternative for breakfast, or topped over yogurt. To make this grain-free, substitute the gluten-free oats for unsweetened coconut flakes.

Serves 10
Preparation: 15 minutes
Cooking: 30–40 minutes

120g/4¼oz/1¼ cups gluten-free oats or unsweetened coconut flakes
60g/2¼oz/¾ cup flaked/sliced almonds
60g/2¼oz/½ cup pecan nuts, chopped
60g/2¼oz/scant ½ cup walnuts, chopped
125g/4½oz/scant 1 cup pumpkin seeds and sunflower seeds
2 tbsp chia seeds
100g/3½oz/¾ cup frozen berries or pitted cherries, defrosted
60g/2¼oz/heaping ½ cup coconut oil, melted, or MCT oil
1 tbsp vanilla extract
1 tbsp medicinal mushroom powder such as lion's mane, cordyceps or chaga
1 tbsp maca powder, or berry powder or beetroot/beet powder (optional)
2 tbsp xylitol or erythritol (optional)

**1** Preheat the oven to 160°C/315°F/Gas 2½ and line two baking sheets with baking parchment. In a large bowl, combine the oats, nuts and seeds, and stir well.

**2** Put the remaining ingredients into a blender or food processor and whiz to make a smooth, thick paste.

**3** Add the paste to the dry ingredients and stir until everything is thoroughly coated – you might find it easier to use your hands.

**4** Spread the granola in a thin layer on the prepared baking sheets, then bake for 30–40 minutes until golden, stirring occasionally to prevent burning. Leave to cool completely, then store in an airtight container for up to 4 weeks.

## Brain Benefits

Superfood powder is included for additional nourishment, whereas maca and cordyceps are both excellent for brain function, as is coconut oil – a fabulous superfuel for the brain.

NUTRITIONAL INFORMATION PER SERVING 419 Kcals, **Protein** 24g,
**Carbohydrates** 23.2g of which sugars 5.2g, **Fat** 23.4g of which saturates 6.9g

# Spinach, Chickpea & Chorizo Hash

Conveniently cooked in one pan, this wonderful Moroccan spiced dish is also delicious made the night before and reheated for a speedy breakfast option. Traditional recipes tend to be carbohydrate heavy because they include potato; this one uses chickpeas and lots of colourful vegetables instead.

Serves 2
Preparation: 15 minutes
Cooking: 10 minutes

2 tsp olive oil
½ red onion, chopped
1 garlic clove, crushed
100g/3½oz cooking chorizo
    sausages, skinned and crumbled
1½ tsp ground allspice
½ tsp za'atar spice mixture
½ tsp smoked paprika
1 tsp ground cumin
½ red pepper/bell pepper,
    deseeded and diced
2 tomatoes, chopped
400g/14oz can chickpeas, drained
    and rinsed
225g/8oz baby spinach leaves
sea salt and ground black pepper

**1** Heat the oil in a large frying pan over a medium heat. Cook the onion and garlic for 2 minutes, then add the chorizo and cook for 5 minutes or until the chorizo is golden and soft.

**2** Add the spices, red pepper/bell pepper, tomatoes and chickpeas, and cook for 2 minutes, mashing up the chickpeas lightly. Add the spinach and stir for 1 minute or until the spinach has wilted. Season with salt and pepper, and serve.

### Brain Benefits
Red pepper/bell pepper and tomatoes are particularly rich in two carotenoids: lycopene and beta-carotene, which help to protect the brain from free-radical damage. In addition to its antioxidant powers, lycopene appears to regulate the genes that influence inflammation and brain growth. Adding fat when eating red peppers and tomatoes helps to improve the body's absorption of the carotenoids.

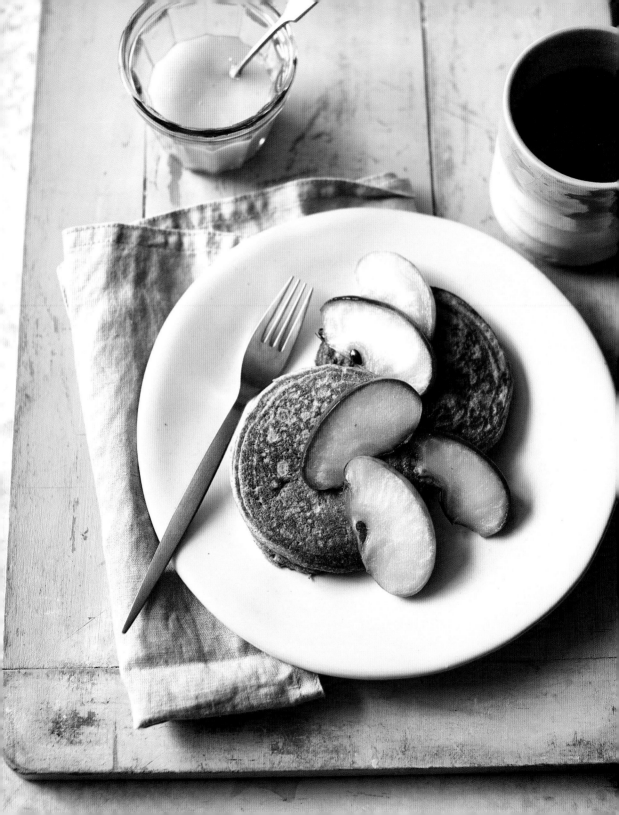

**V** NUTRITIONAL INFORMATION PER SERVING 373 Kcals, **Protein** 9.5g, **Carbohydrates** 46.5g of which sugars 4.9g, **Fat** 15.1g of which saturates 9g

# Caramel Apple Pancakes

These simple, grain-free pancakes are fabulous hot out of the pan, or cold as a snack. The caramel sauce is optional – if you want to keep the calories and carbohydrates lower, omit it but top with coconut or Greek yogurt mixed with a little cinnamon. For a dairy-free option, use coconut oil rather than butter.

Serves 3
Preparation: 20 minutes
Cooking: 12 minutes

3 eggs
100ml/3½fl oz/scant ½ cup almond
    milk
1 tsp vanilla extract
50g/1¾oz/scant ½ cup coconut
    flour
50g/1¾oz/scant ½ cup tapioca flour
1 tsp baking powder
4 tbsp bicarbonate of soda
1 tsp ground cinnamon
1 tbsp coconut oil or olive oil, plus
    extra for greasing
1 medium apple, thinly sliced

FOR THE CARAMEL
2 tsp arrowroot powder
150ml/5fl oz/⅔ cup coconut milk
50g/1¾oz/¼ cup xylitol or
    erythritol
1 tbsp unsalted butter or coconut
    oil

**1** To make the caramel, mix the arrowroot with 2 tablespoons of the milk to make a paste. Put the xylitol and the remaining milk in a saucepan over a medium-low heat and gradually heat it so that the xylitol dissolves. Add the butter, and bring to a gentle boil. Boil for 5 minutes or until the mixture begins to reduce and thicken slightly, stirring constantly. Pour in the arrowroot mixture and gently simmer for 1 minute to allow the mixture to thicken. Leave to cool. Store in the refrigerator for up to 1 week.

**2** Put the eggs into a blender or food processor and add the milk, vanilla, flours, baking powder, bicarbonate of soda and cinnamon, then whiz to form a thick batter. Heat the oil in a frying pan over a medium heat and add the apple. Cook gently for 2–3 minutes until the apple is softened. Leave to one side.

**3** Add a little more oil to the pan, if needed, for greasing. Spoon a few spoonfuls of the batter into the pan to make small pancakes, and cook for 2 minutes on each side until golden. Repeat with the remaining batter to make 6 pancakes. Serve the pancakes with the apple and drizzled with the caramel.

**Brain Benefits**
The antioxidant plant compound quercetin in apples has been shown to protect brain cells from free-radical damage. Apples are also rich in the soluble fibre pectin, and polyphenols which support the growth of our beneficial gut bacteria.

**V** NUTRITIONAL INFORMATION PER MUFFIN 195 Kcals, **Protein** 6.6g, **Carbohydrates** 10.7g of which sugars 0.6g, **Fat** 13.8g of which saturates 2.7g

# Feta, Herb & Olive Muffins

Mediterranean-inspired, these muffins are full of flavour with a crunch at the top. You could also add some chopped sun-dried tomatoes to the mixture, if you like.

Makes 12 muffins

Preparation: 15 minutes

Cooking: 15–20 minutes

100g/3½oz/1 cup ground almonds

150g/5½oz/scant 1¼ cups gluten-free flour

½ tsp sea salt

½ tsp ground black pepper

2 tsp baking powder

2 tbsp parsley leaves, finely chopped

1 tbsp finely chopped tarragon leaves or other herbs, to taste

3 eggs

2 tbsp milk or coconut milk/almond milk

50ml/1¾fl oz/scant ¼ cup extra virgin olive oil

100g/3½oz feta cheese, crumbled

100g/3½oz/1 cup pitted black olives, chopped

30g/1oz/¼ cup pumpkin seeds, to decorate

**1** Preheat the oven to 180°C/350°F/Gas 4 and line a 12-cup muffin tray with paper cases. Put the almonds and flour into a food processor and add the salt, pepper, baking powder and herbs, then whiz to combine.

**2** Add the eggs, milk and oil, and whiz to form a batter. Stir in the feta cheese and olives. (Alternatively, mix well in a bowl using an electric hand whisk/beater.) Spoon the batter into the prepared muffin tray, then scatter a few pumpkin seeds over the tops.

**3** Bake for 15–20 minutes until a skewer comes out clean. Leave the muffins to cool in the tray, then turn out to serve.

**Brain Benefits**

More than just a garnish, parsley contains plentiful amounts of brain-supporting nutrients. It is also a good source of vitamin K, which might play a role in the treatment and possible prevention of Alzheimer's disease by limiting neuronal damage in the brain. Furthermore, it is rich in protective antioxidants and vitamin C.

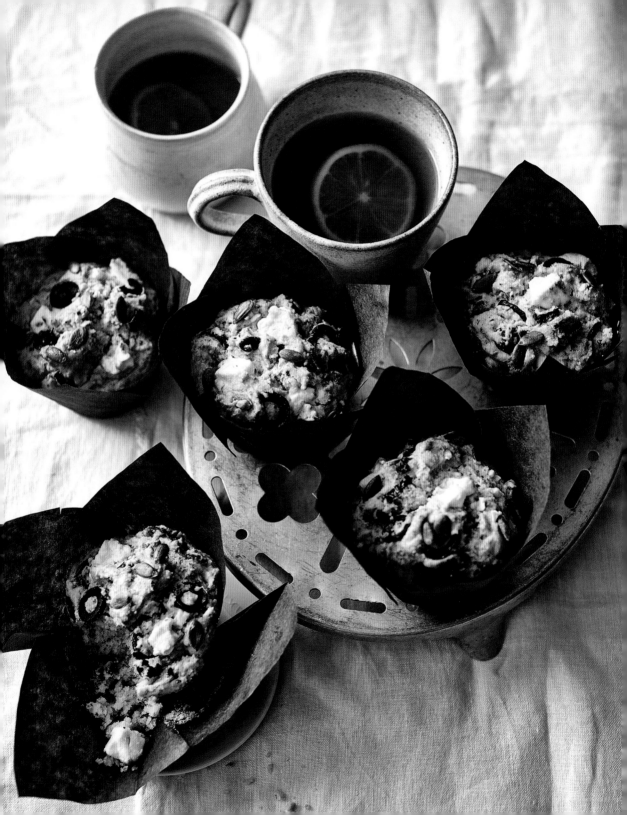

# The Breakfast Loaf

A no-yeast bread that is perfect warm or toasted, this seeded loaf is an ideal replacement for conventional breads. It uses ground almonds as its base with yogurt or kefir to help keep the loaf lovely and moist. Once you have made your loaf, there is a whole host of different recipes that you can try – some are perfect for a long, lazy brunch while others are a quick, grab-and-go morning snack.

## Breakfast Seeded Bread

  NUTRITIONAL INFORMATION PER SLICE 249 Kcals, **Protein** 9.8g, **Carbohydrates** 9.1g of which sugars 1.4g, **Fat** 19g of which saturates 2.2g

MAKES 1 x 2lb/900g loaf, 12 slices   PREPARATION: 15 minutes   COOKING: 40 minutes

✛3 tbsp olive oil or melted coconut oil, plus extra for greasing ✛250g/9oz/2½ cups ground almonds ✛2 tbsp chia seeds ✛½ tsp salt ✛½ tsp bicarbonate of soda ✛1 tsp baking powder ✛70g/2½oz/½ cup arrowroot powder ✛ 5 eggs ✛1 tsp apple cider vinegar ✛4 tbsp yogurt or Kefir (page 63) ✛60g/2¼oz/scant ½ cup mixed seeds, plus extra for topping

**1** Preheat the oven to 180°C/350°F/Gas 4 and lightly grease and line a 2lb/900g loaf pan with baking parchment. Put the almonds in a food processor and add the chia seeds, salt, bicarbonate of soda, baking powder and arrowroot, and whiz briefly to mix.
**2** Add the oil, eggs, vinegar and yogurt, and whiz until smooth. Pulse, or stir, in the seeds. Spoon the mixture into the prepared loaf pan and smooth the top. Scatter some extra seeds over the top.
**3** Bake for 40 minutes or until a skewer inserted into the centre comes out clean. Leave to cool in the pan for 10 minutes, then turn out onto a wire rack to cool completely. Serve in slices. The sliced loaf can be frozen: open-freeze the slices until firm, then pack into bags and store in the freezer for up to 3 months.

### Brain Benefits
Sunflower seeds are rich in vitamin E, the main fat-soluble antioxidant, which helps to protect the brain from free-radical damage. They are also rich in magnesium, an essential mineral for the production of many neurotransmitters and can help to prevent migraine headaches.

## VARIATIONS

➤ Make this savoury by stirring in ½ grated onion or chopped spring onion/scallion and some chopped fresh or dried herbs. You can also add grated carrot, courgette/zucchini or sweet potato.

➤ For a sweeter option, substitute 30g/1oz of the almonds for raw cacao powder and add 2 tablespoons granulated stevia, or xylitol or erythritol, to taste.

## HEALTHY TOPPINGS TO TRY

➤ **PESTO GREEN EGGS**
Use a fork to mix 4 eggs with a pinch of salt. Melt a little coconut oil in a frying pan set over a medium heat, then pour in the egg mixture. Gently stir with a wooden spoon to scramble. Add and stir in 2 tablespoons pesto (pages 152–3) and heat through. Serve on toast.

➤ **SMASHED AVOCADO**
Put ½ ripe avocado in a bowl with a splash of tamari soy sauce and 2 teaspoons white miso paste. Mash with a fork until smooth. Stir in ½ chopped tomato, if you like. Spread on bread.

➤ **KIMCHI WITH POACHED EGG OR SMOKED SALMON**
Spread kimchi or sauerkraut on toast and add a poached egg or smoked salmon.

➤ **BROCCOLI WITH CHEESE**
Put cooked broccoli florets on top of bread and top with grated cheese, then grill/broil.

➤ **MARINARA SARDINES**
Drizzle a little olive oil over bread or toast. Spread with Ketchup (page 70) or passata and top with canned sardines lightly mashed with a fork. Heat through under the grill/broiler.

➤ **FETA CHEESE WITH MINT & AVOCADO**
Mash ½ ripe avocado with 30g/1oz crumbled feta cheese and some chopped fresh mint with a dash of lemon juice. Spread on bread.

➤ **SAUERKRAUT AND APPLE**
Top toast with sauerkraut and slices of apple or pear.

➤ Also try: Homemade Nut Butter (page 74), Sugar-Free Strawberry Butter (page 75), Chocolate Nut Spread (page 75) and Smashed Lemon Chickpea Spread (page 209) to top bread.

# Savoury Waffles with Creamy Mushrooms

Make up some of these waffles for a brunch or light lunch. They can be made in advance and kept in the fridge for up to 2 days, making them ideal as a grab-and-go breakfast option. This recipe is dairy-free, but you can add a couple of spoonfuls of grated Parmesan cheese to the batter, if you like.

Makes 4 large waffles

Preparation: 15 minutes

Cooking: 10 minutes

100–125ml/3½–4fl oz/scant ½ cup–
  ½ cup almond milk

5 eggs

100g/3½oz/scant 1 cup almond
  flour (not ground almonds)

30g/1oz/¼ cup coconut flour

3 tbsp arrowroot powder

1 tsp bicarbonate of soda

¼ tsp ground turmeric

2 tbsp nutritional yeast flakes
  optional (or use grated
  Parmesan cheese)

2 tbsp extra virgin olive oil, or MCT
  oil or coconut oil, plus 2 tsp olive
  oil and extra for greasing

2 tsp apple cider vinegar

2 garlic cloves, crushed

1 tomato, chopped

8 button or chestnut mushrooms,
  thinly sliced

100ml/3½fl oz/scant ½ cup full-fat
  canned coconut milk

sea salt and ground black pepper

1 Pour 100ml/3½fl oz/scant ½ cup almond milk into a high-speed blender or food processor and add the eggs, flours, arrowroot, bicarbonate of soda, ¼ teaspoon salt, turmeric, yeast flakes, the 2 tablespoons oil and the vinegar. Whiz to form a smooth, thick batter, adding a little more milk if needed.

2 Grease a waffle iron. Pour the batter into the waffle iron and cook for 5 minutes or according to the manufacturer's directions. Repeat with the remaining batter.

3 Meanwhile, to make the creamy mushrooms, heat the 2 teaspoons oil in a frying pan over a low heat and cook the garlic and tomato for 2 minutes, stirring occasionally. Add the mushrooms and fry for another 2 minutes or until soft. Pour in the milk and simmer for 2 minutes to thicken the sauce. Season with salt and pepper and serve with the waffles.

### Brain Benefits

Both edible and medicinal mushrooms are known to support nerve and brain health. They are a great source of B vitamins, fibre, antioxidants and polysaccharides, including beta-glucans – compounds which are known for their immune-supporting benefits.

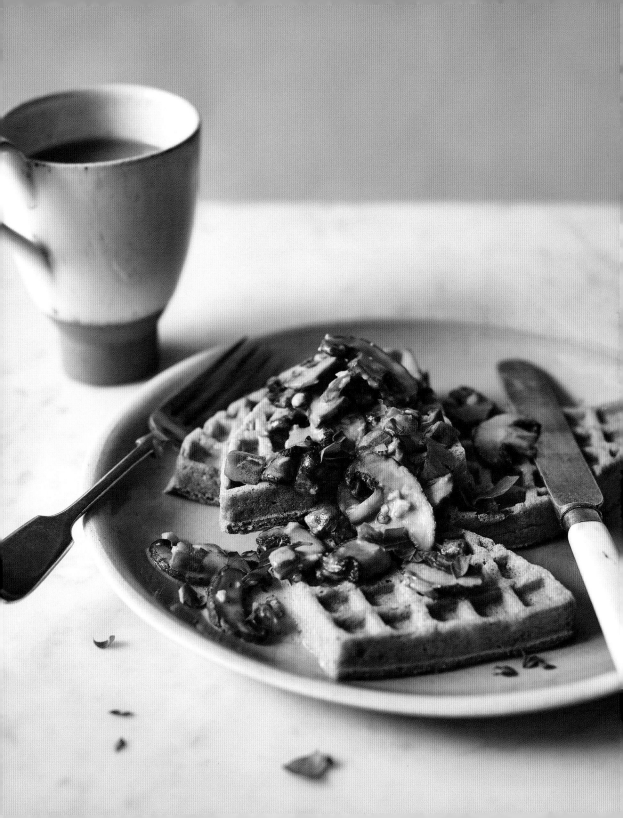

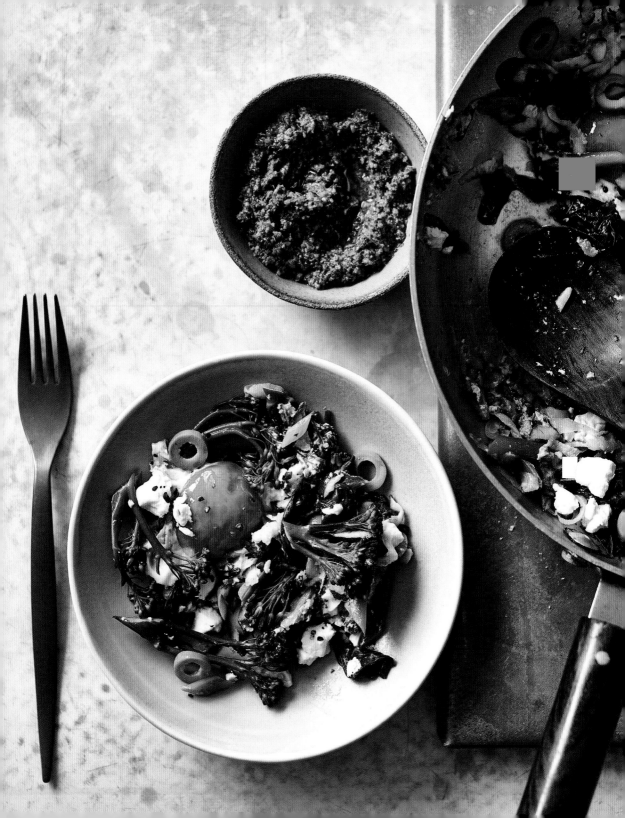

**P** **V**

ACCORDING
TO CHOICES

NUTRITIONAL INFORMATION PER SERVING (using 1 egg per person) 196 Kcals,
**Protein** 9.5g, **Carbohydrates** 2.7g of which sugars 1.9g, **Fat** 15.8g of which saturates 6.2g

# Green Shakshuka

You can serve this vibrant, fresh-tasting breakfast dish as a speedy lunch option too, as it takes just minutes to make and is sustaining. It's also a delicious way to use up leftover veggies.

Serves 2
Preparation: 15 minutes, plus
    making the pesto
Cooking: 12 minutes

1 tbsp coconut oil or olive oil
3 spring onions/scallions, chopped
1 grated courgette/zucchini (or
    use leftover cooked courgette/
    zucchini)
100g/3½oz/2 cups broccoli florets
    (either raw or leftover cooked)
½ tsp ground cumin
a pinch of dried chilli/hot pepper
    flakes
juice of ½ lemon
1 large handful of baby spinach
    leaves or other leafy greens
2 tbsp pesto (pages 152–3)
2–4 eggs (according to appetite)
30g/1oz feta cheese, crumbled
    (optional)
30g/1oz/⅓ cup pitted olives
    (optional), chopped
sea salt and ground black pepper

**1** Heat the oil in a large frying pan over a medium heat. Add the spring onions/scallions, raw courgette/zucchini and broccoli florets. (If using leftover cooked vegetables, add these a little later.) Cook for 5 minutes or until the vegetables are softened. Add the cumin and dried chilli/hot pepper flakes, lemon juice, spinach and leftover cooked vegetables, if using. Cook for 1–2 minutes until the greens have wilted. Stir in the pesto and season with salt and pepper.

**2** Create little dents in the mixture and crack in the eggs. Cover the pan with a lid and cook for 5 minutes or until the eggs are set. Scatter over the cheese and olives, if you like, and serve.

**Brain Benefits**
Eggs are a fabulous brain food, packed with vitamin B12 and choline. Vitamin B12 helps the body to fight against brain shrinkage, whereas choline is an important building block of the brain cells and for the production of acetylcholine, our memory neurotransmitter.

# Indian Spiced Omelette

Here is a delicious spicy twist on the traditional omelette, stuffed with green chilli, fresh coriander/
cilantro and turmeric. A little homemade tomato Ketchup (page 70) complements the favours very well.

Serves 2

Preparation: 10 minutes

Cooking: 3 minutes

1 tbsp coconut oil

1 small onion, finely chopped

1 small tomato, finely chopped

1 green chilli, deseeded and finely
chopped

4 eggs

½ tsp ground turmeric

2 tbsp coriander/cilantro leaves,
chopped

a squeeze of lemon juice

sea salt and ground black pepper

**1** Heat the oil in a frying pan over a medium heat and add the onion, tomato and chilli. Cook for 1 minute.

**2** In a small bowl, whisk the eggs lightly with the turmeric. Season with salt and pepper, and stir in the coriander/cilantro.

**3** Pour the egg mixture into the pan and give it a quick swirl to distribute it evenly across the pan. Cook for 1 minute until it sets and is light brown and slightly crisp around the edge. Flip the omelette over and cook the other side for 1 minute. Fold the omelette over and tip it out of the pan. Squeeze over a little lemon juice and serve.

### Brain Benefits

Coconut oil and black pepper aid the absorption of curcumin, the active component in turmeric known for its many brain-boosting benefits.

**P** NUTRITIONAL INFORMATION PER SERVING 273 Kcals, **Protein** 26.4g,
**Carbohydrates** 18.6g of which sugars 10.9g, **Fat** 9.5g of which saturates 5.3g

# Chilli Breakfast Bowl

This might seem to be a strange breakfast option, but a bowl of warming chilli with liver is an excellent way to nourish the brain and kick-start the day. Using turkey provides plenty of protein without raising inflammation and it perfectly complements the chicken livers.

Serves 2
Preparation: 15 minutes
Cooking: 25 minutes

1 tbsp coconut oil
½ onion, finely diced
2 mushrooms, diced
½ sweet potato, diced
2 garlic cloves, crushed
100g/3½oz chicken livers, finely
    diced
150g/5½oz/⅔ cup lean minced/
    ground turkey
½ tsp dried oregano
½ tsp ground cumin
½ tsp ground cinnamon
½ tsp chilli powder
400g/14oz can chopped tomatoes
    or passata
1 large handful of chopped kale
chopped coriander/cilantro leaves,
    diced avocado and tomato,
    to serve

**1** Heat the oil in a large frying pan over a medium heat and add the onion, mushrooms, sweet potato and garlic. Cook for 5 minutes or until the sweet potato begins to soften.

**2** Add the livers, turkey, oregano and spices, stir well and cook for 4 minutes or until the meat starts to turn golden, stirring frequently.

**3** Add the remaining ingredients, mix well, then cover and simmer for 15 minutes or until the turkey is cooked through. Serve with the coriander/cilantro, avocado and tomato scattered on top.

### Brain Benefits
Liver is a great source of vitamin A, the B vitamins and iron, making it an ideal fatigue fighter. If you can, choose organic or grass-fed meat, which is free from toxic contamination.

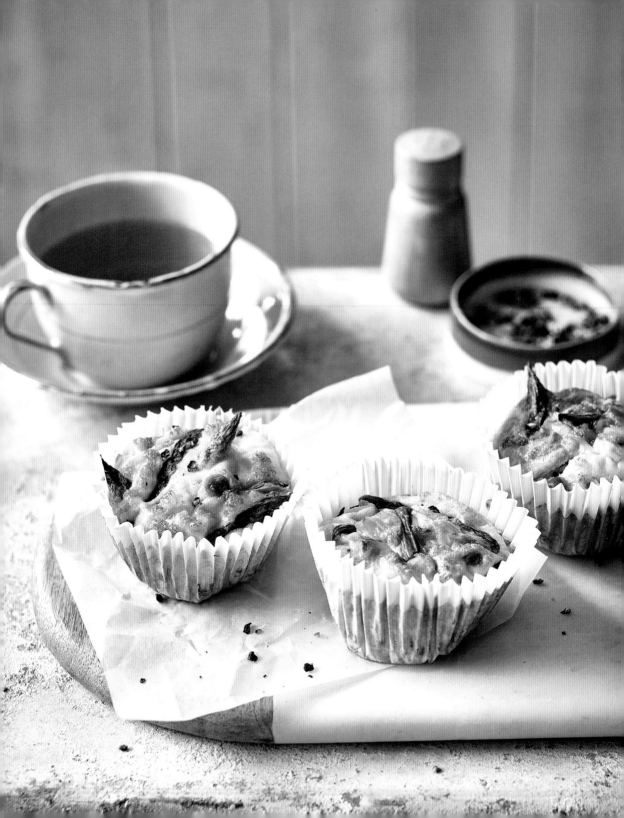

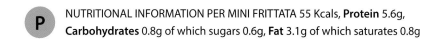

NUTRITIONAL INFORMATION PER MINI FRITTATA 55 Kcals, **Protein** 5.6g, **Carbohydrates** 0.8g of which sugars 0.6g, **Fat** 3.1g of which saturates 0.8g

# Asparagus & Salmon Mini Frittatas

These colourful savoury muffins are easy to make and are delicious served warm for breakfast or cold for lunch with a salad.

**Makes 8 mini frittatas**
**Preparation: 15 minutes**
**Cooking: 23 minutes**

125g/4½oz asparagus
1 handful of frozen peas
2 spring onions/scallions, chopped
60g/2¼oz smoked salmon, cut into
    small strips
4 eggs, beaten
sea salt and ground black pepper

**1** Preheat the oven to 200°C/400°F/Gas 6 and grease and line 8 cups of a muffin tray with paper muffin cases. Blanch the asparagus in a saucepan of boiling salted water for 2–3 minutes until just soft. Drain, then cut into 1cm/½in pieces using scissors.

**2** Divide the asparagus, peas, spring onions/scallions and smoked salmon among the paper cases – they should be three-quarters full. Beat the eggs in a jug/pitcher with some salt and pepper, then pour into the paper cases.

**3** Bake in the centre of the oven for 20 minutes or until the muffins are golden and just firm in the centre. Leave to cool for 5 minutes before removing them from the tray. Serve hot or cold.

**Brain Benefits**
Asparagus is rich in folate and other B vitamins, which can help to maintain a healthy homocysteine level (see page 9) and support the production of neurotransmitters to boost mood. Asparagus is also a good source of vitamin A – critical for enabling plasticity in the adult brain – which helps the brain to adapt and grow during learning.

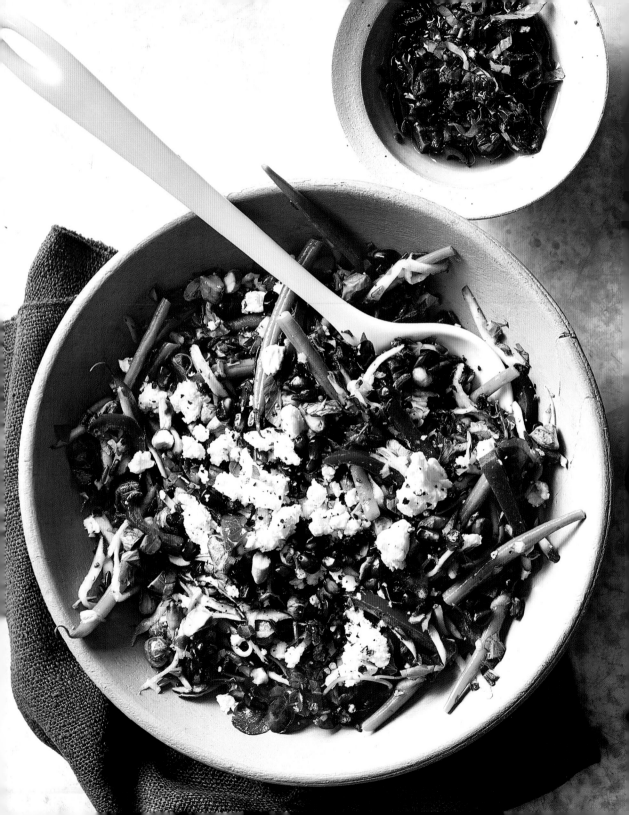

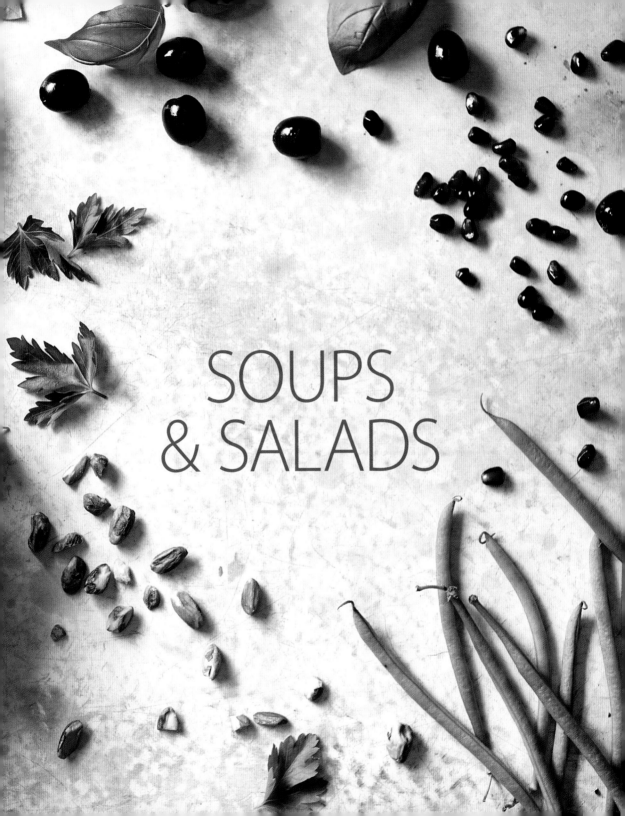

SOUPS
& SALADS

**V** **VE** NUTRITIONAL INFORMATION PER SERVING 206 Kcals, **Protein** 3.9g, **Carbohydrates** 23.7g of which sugars 14.1g, **Fat** 9.5g of which saturates 6.5g

# Squash & Apple Soup with Miso Butter

Roasted squash or pumpkin is naturally sweet and comforting and a perfect autumn food. The miso butter adds to the full flavour of the soup and is equally delicious served over baked fish or seafood.

Serves 2
Preparation: 15 minutes
Cooking: 20 minutes

15g/½oz/1 tbsp coconut oil
1 onion, chopped
4 garlic cloves, crushed
300g/10½oz butternut squash
 or pumpkin, peeled, deseeded
 and cut into 2cm/¾in cubes
1 eating apple, cored and chopped
500ml/17fl oz/2 cups vegetable
 stock or chicken stock
1 tbsp white miso paste
2 tsp unsalted butter, softened, or
 coconut oil
sea salt and ground black pepper
pumpkin seeds (optional), to
 garnish

**1** Heat the oil in a large, heavy saucepan over a medium heat. Add the onion and garlic, and cook gently for 2–3 minutes until the onion is soft.

**2** Add the butternut squash, apple and stock. Bring to the boil, then lower the heat and simmer for 15 minutes, or until the squash is very tender.

**3** Meanwhile, in a bowl, beat together 1 tablespoon of the miso paste with a little black pepper and the softened butter until completely smooth.

**4** Add the remaining miso to the squash mixture. Using a blender or food processor, whiz the soup until smooth and creamy. Season with salt and pepper to taste. Ladle the soup into bowls and top with a dollop of miso butter and pumpkin seeds, if you like.

### Brain Benefits
Squash and pumpkin are packed with antioxidants, particularly the carotenoids, which, together with their wealth of vitamins, including B vitamins, plus iron, magnesium and copper, appear to be particularly important for cognitive function. The fat in this recipe also enhances the absorption of the carotenoids. Apple is a great source of prebiotic fibre to support the growth of beneficial bacteria in the gut.

NUTRITIONAL INFORMATION PER SERVING 309 Kcals, **Protein** 17.1g, **Carbohydrates** 22.1g of which sugars 17.6g, **Fat** 13.9g of which saturates 6.8g

# Broccoli Tahini Cream Soup

With ingredients that are perfect for cleansing the body and brain, this creamy soup is full of goodness as well as being easy to make and satisfying.

Serves 2
Preparation: 15 minutes
Cooking: 18 minutes

1 tbsp coconut oil
1 small onion, chopped
2 garlic cloves, crushed
1cm/½in piece of root ginger,
  peeled and grated
a pinch of dried chilli/hot pepper
  flakes
1½ heads of broccoli, cut into
  florets
400g/14oz can full-fat coconut milk
200ml/7fl oz/scant 1 cup vegetable
  stock
sea salt and ground black pepper

FOR THE TOPPING
1 tbsp tahini
2 tbsp Greek yogurt or coconut
  yogurt
1 tbsp lemon juice
1 tbsp chopped coriander/cilantro
  leaves

**1** Heat the oil in a large saucepan over a medium heat and cook the onion, garlic and ginger for 3–4 minutes until the onion begins to soften.

**2** Add the dried chilli/hot pepper flakes, broccoli, milk and vegetable stock. Bring to the boil, then reduce the heat and simmer gently for 10 minutes or until the broccoli is just soft. Season with salt and pepper to taste.

**3** Meanwhile, make the topping. Mix together the tahini, yogurt and lemon juice with 1 tablespoon water or enough to form a thick sauce. Ladle the soup into bowls and swirl in the tahini cream, then scatter over chopped coriander/cilantro leaves and serve.

**Brain Benefits**
Adding tahini to the soup boosts the calcium and magnesium content as well as providing essential fatty acids, which can be useful for de-stressing the body and aiding relaxation.

**P** NUTRITIONAL INFORMATION PER SERVING 294 Kcals, **Protein** 35.8g, **Carbohydrates** 5g of which sugars 3.9g, **Fat** 13.7g of which saturates 5.7g

# Meatball & Kale Soup

This light broth-based soup makes a warming, comforting and appetizing lunch. The bite-size meatballs are tasty and rich and are combined with health-giving kale as a meal in a bowl.

Serves 2
Preparation: 15 minutes
Cooking: 20 minutes

1 tbsp coconut oil
1 red onion, cut in half and thinly
    sliced
1 garlic clove, crushed
100g/3½oz kale, chopped
1 tomato, deseeded and chopped
500ml/17fl oz/2 cups chicken stock
chopped parsley leaves, to serve

FOR THE MEATBALLS
200g/7oz/scant 1 cup lean minced/
    ground turkey
1 egg yolk
1 tbsp ground almonds
1 tbsp Parmesan cheese (optional)
1 tbsp chopped parsley leaves
a pinch of sea salt and ground black
    pepper
coconut oil, for frying

**1** Heat the coconut oil in a large saucepan over a medium heat. Add the onion and garlic, and cook over a low heat for 10 minutes or until the onion is golden.

**2** Meanwhile, to make the meatballs, put all the ingredients, except the oil, in a large bowl and mix well. Using your hands, roll the mixture into walnut-size balls. Heat a small amount of oil in a frying pan and cook the meatballs for 3–4 minutes, turning regularly, until browned and crisp.

**3** Add the kale, tomato and stock to the saucepan and bring to the boil, then reduce the heat. Add the meatballs and simmer for 3–4 minutes until the kale is tender and the meatballs are cooked through. Ladle into bowls and scatter over parsley to serve.

## Brain Benefits

Kale is a nutrient-dense cruciferous vegetable, rich with B vitamins and magnesium, which are important for mental performance. The turkey provides essential protein and the amino acid tryptophan to support a healthy mood.

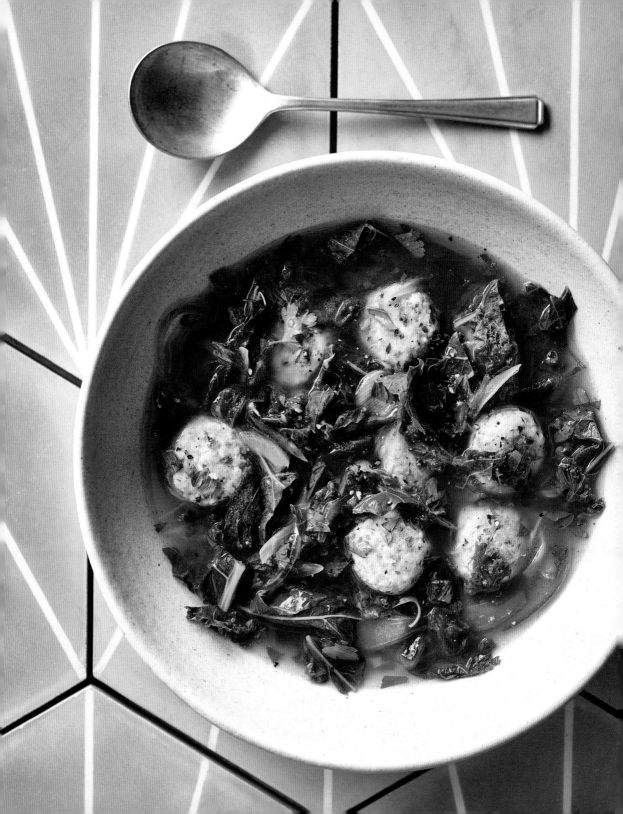

NUTRITIONAL INFORMATION PER SERVING 349 Kcals, **Protein** 36.5g, **Carbohydrates** 26.1g of which sugars 10.9g, **Fat** 9.3g of which saturates 1.9g

# Chicken Enchilada Soup

This delicious one-pot Mexican-style soup is rich with flavour and fibre from the addition of black beans. If you have a slow cooker, you can add all the ingredients to the crock and cook on Low for 6–8 hours until the chicken is tender.

Serves 2
Preparation: 10 minutes
Cooking: 45 minutes

400g/14oz can chopped tomatoes
300ml/10½fl oz/1¼ cups chicken
   stock
200g/7oz skinless chicken breasts
½ onion, diced
½ red pepper/bell pepper,
   deseeded and diced
1 celery stalk, finely diced
½ red chilli, deseeded and finely
   chopped
1 garlic clove, crushed
1 tsp chilli powder or taco
   seasoning
1 tsp ground cumin
¼ tsp smoked paprika
½ x 400g/14oz can black beans,
   drained and rinsed
1 tbsp chopped coriander/cilantro
   leaves
½ avocado, pitted, skinned and
   sliced
sea salt and ground black pepper
1 handful of gluten-free corn
   tortillas, to serve

**1** Preheat the oven to 170°C/325°F/Gas 3. Put the chopped tomatoes and stock in a flameproof casserole.

**2** Put the chicken in the casserole and put the onion, red pepper/ bell pepper, celery, chilli and garlic on top of the chicken. Stir in the chilli powder, cumin and paprika, and add the beans. Season with salt and pepper.

**3** Cover the casserole and bring to the boil on the hob/stovetop over a medium-high heat. Transfer to the oven and cook for 40 minutes or until the chicken is tender. Use a fork to shred the chicken and divide it among serving bowls, then spoon the soup over. Top with the coriander/cilantro and avocado, and serve with corn tortillas.

**Brain Benefits**

Chicken is a good source of lean protein, and also contains dietary choline and vitamins B6 and B12 to help maintain healthy homocysteine levels (see page 9). Choline and the B vitamins have been shown to play important roles in healthy cognition and provide neuro-protective benefits. Choline is an essential building block in acetylcholine, a brain chemical that helps memory.

NUTRITIONAL INFORMATION PER SERVING 234 Kcals, **Protein** 34.8g, **Carbohydrates** 7.6g of which sugars 5.9g, **Fat** 6.4g of which saturates 4.3g

# Jjamppong

This Korean spiced seafood soup is rich with vegetables and shellfish and goes well with Kimchi (page 68). Rather than using traditional noodles, courgette/zucchini ribbons keep the carbohydrates lower. If you cannot find gochugaru, use smoked dried chilli/hot pepper flakes or chilli paste instead.

Serves 2
Preparation: 15 minutes, plus 15
    minutes soaking
Cooking: 12 minutes

2 dried shiitake mushrooms
500ml/17fl oz/2 cups chicken stock
350g/12oz raw mixed seafood, such
    as shelled prawns/shrimp, squid,
    mussels in shells, clams in shells,
    or 300g/10½oz cooked shellfish
1 tbsp coconut oil
2 spring onions/scallions, finely
    chopped
1 garlic clove, crushed
5mm/¼in piece of root ginger,
    peeled and finely grated
2 tsp gochugaru (Korean dried
    chilli/hot pepper flakes), smoked
    dried chilli/hot pepper flakes or
    chilli paste
½ Chinese cabbage, shredded
2 tbsp tomato purée/paste
1 tbsp tamari soy sauce
1 tbsp mirin
1 courgette/zucchini, spiralized or
    cut into long ribbons
1 handful of baby spinach leaves
sea salt and ground black pepper

**1** Put the shiitake mushrooms in a small bowl and pour over 100ml/3½fl oz/scant ½ cup boiling water. Leave to soak for 15 minutes. Remove the mushrooms and strain the soaking liquid into the chicken stock. Leave to one side. Slice the mushrooms.

**2** If using seafood in shells, scrub the shells and discard any that remain open after being sharply tapped. Scrape off the beards from the mussels.

**3** Heat the oil in a large saucepan and add the spring onions, garlic, ginger, dried chilli/hot pepper flakes, mushrooms and Chinese cabbage. Stir-fry for 2 minutes. Pour the chicken stock into the pan and add the tomato purée/paste. Bring to the boil.

**4** If using shellfish in shells, add them to the pan. Bring to the boil, then simmer gently for 5 minutes or until the shellfish have opened and cooked. Discard any shells that remain closed. If using cooked shellfish, add them to the pan and cook for 2 minutes to heat through.

**5** Add the tamari and mirin, courgette/zucchini and spinach, and heat until the spinach has wilted. Season with salt and pepper, and serve.

### Brain Benefits

Prawns/shrimp are a superb brain-boosting food, containing plenty of vitamin B12 and omega-3 fatty acids, both of which have been associated with protecting the ageing brain from cognitive decline.

**V** NUTRITIONAL INFORMATION PER SERVING 234 Kcals, **Protein** 22.3g, **Carbohydrates** 12.8g of which sugars 5.4g, **Fat** 8.2g of which saturates 0.8g

# Vegetarian Hot & Sour Soup

Fresh turmeric is not traditional in hot-and-sour soup, but is a tasty way to include more anti-inflammatory spices in your diet. Tempeh is preferable to tofu here, because it is fermented and is easier to digest, but if you are unable to find it, use tofu or use 2–3 eggs instead of one.

Serves 2

Preparation: 15 minutes, plus
    15 minutes soaking

Cooking: 11 minutes

1 small handful of dried seaweed,
    such as nori, dulse, wakame
500ml/17fl oz/2 cups vegetable stock
1cm/½in piece of root ginger, peeled
    and grated
1cm/½in piece of turmeric root,
    peeled and finely grated or ½ tsp
    ground turmeric
½ red chilli, deseeded and chopped
2 spring onions/scallions, sliced
2 shiitake mushrooms, thinly sliced
1 small carrot, cut into matchsticks
225g/8oz can bamboo shoots, drained
1 tbsp mirin
1 tbsp tamari soy sauce
1 tbsp rice vinegar
1 handful of bean sprouts
150g/5½oz tempeh or firm tofu, cut
    into small cubes
2 tsp white miso paste
1 tbsp cornflour/cornstarch
1 egg, beaten
1 spring onion/scallion, chopped,
    to garnish

**1** Put the seaweed in a small bowl and cover with water. Leave to soak for 15 minutes, then drain.

**2** Pour the stock into a saucepan over a medium-high heat and add the seaweed, ginger, turmeric, chilli, spring onions/scallions, mushrooms and carrot, then bring to the boil. Reduce the heat and simmer for 5 minutes or until the vegetables are tender. Add the bamboo shoots, mirin, tamari, vinegar, bean sprouts, tempeh and miso paste.

**3** Put the cornflour/cornstarch in a bowl and add 3 tablespoons water. Mix well and add to the soup. Stir until it begins to thicken, about 5 minutes. Slowly drizzle the egg into the soup to form ribbons, stirring as you pour. Ladle the soup into bowls and garnish scattered with the spring onion, then serve.

## Brain Benefits

Seaweed is a rich source of trace minerals including iodine, which is essential for brain cognition and IQ. Miso is a salty fermented paste plentiful in beneficial bacteria to support a healthy gut.

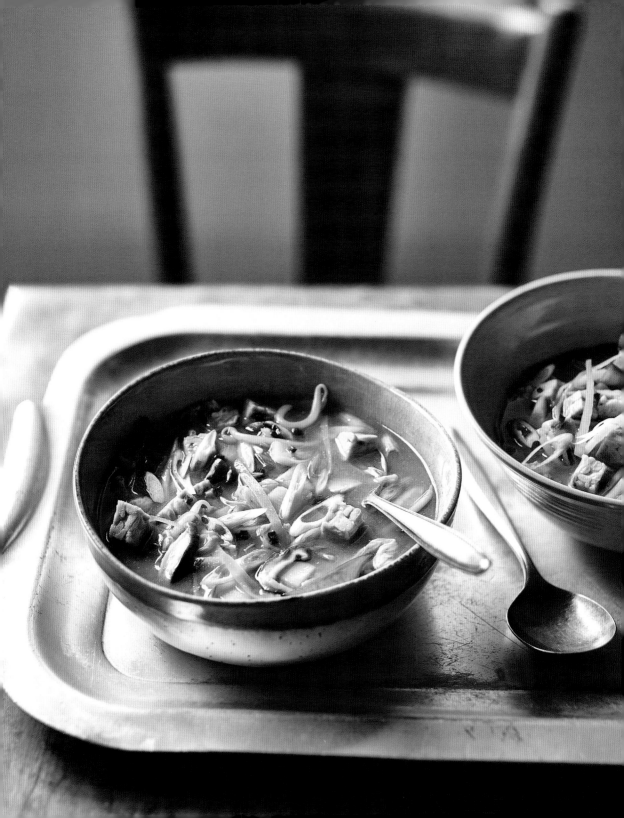

# Nourish Bowls

Whether it's noodles in Japan, bibimbap in Korea or bowl food derived from the Swedish hygge, many cultures have traditional one-bowl meals, which are immensely nourishing. Nourish bowls, as I like to call them, are also speedy and simple to create, particularly if you make use of raw veggies or leftover cooked vegetables in the refrigerator. The key is to create a balanced bowl with your combination of vegetables, lean protein and healthy fats. Keep it colourful and bold with plenty of flavours. The result is a complete meal to energize the body.

## HOW TO BUILD YOUR NOURISH BOWL

➤ **COLOURFUL VEGGIES.** Aim for half the bowl or 3 servings of colourful vegetables – whether raw or cooked. One serving is 1 large handful leafy greens or a small handful (80g/2¾oz) of other chopped vegetables. This is a good basis to support detoxification, magnesium and B vitamins.

➤ **LEAN PROTEIN.** At least a quarter of your bowl should be protein. A serving is 2 eggs, a palm-sized portion of lean meat (poultry, beef, lamb or pork) or fish (including shellfish), 130g/4¾oz/1 cup cooked beans or 50g/1¾oz/¼ cup cottage cheese.

➤ **HEALTHY FATS.** Whether it's a handful of nuts and seeds, some avocado, olives or a dressing, the healthy fats will give your brain much-needed nourishment.

➤ **OPTIONAL SLOW-RELEASE CARBS.** For a more energizing bowl, keep slow-release carbs low (about a fist size, cooked). These could be roasted root vegetables, grated beetroot/beet, cooked quinoa or red rice. If you are using beans and pulses for protein, be aware that these contain a reasonable amount of carbohydrate as well, so you might not need any additional carb.

➤ **OTHER ADDITIONS.** Be inventive – think probiotic-rich foods to nourish the gut and the brain, such as kimchi, sauerkraut, homemade pickles, yogurt, miso and kefir in dressings (see pages 60–69). Add a turmeric dressing for anti-inflammatory benefits, or use MCT oil in the dressing or flaxseed oil for additional omega-3 fats. I also like to blend antioxidant powders, such as medicinal mushrooms or green superfoods, into the dressings.

# Spicy Chickpea Bowl with Turmeric Dressing

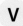 **V**

NUTRITIONAL INFORMATION PER SERVING 334 Kcals, **Protein** 12.7g,
**Carbohydrates** 37.8g of which sugars 14.2g, **Fat** 11.6g of which saturates 2.6g

SERVES 2   PREPARATION: 15 minutes, plus making the Chickpea Crunchies   COOKING: 28 minutes

✛1 red pepper/bell pepper, deseeded and cut into chunks ✛1 small sweet potato, cut into chunks ✛1 small red
onion, cut into wedges ✛2 tbsp olive oil ✛1 head of broccoli, cut into florets ✛2 large handfuls of kale, chopped
✛1 × quantity Garlic & Turmeric Chickpea Crunchies (see page 210) ✛2 tbsp pomegranate seeds or goji berries
✛salt and ground black pepper  TURMERIC DRESSING ✛½ tsp ground turmeric ✛2 tsp tahini ✛2 tbsp Greek
yogurt or coconut yogurt ✛1 tsp xylitol or erythritol, or to taste ✛zest and juice of ½ lemon

**1** Preheat the oven to 200°C/400°F/Gas 6. Put the
red pepper/bell pepper on a baking sheet and add
the sweet potato and onion. Drizzle with a little of
the oil, and toss to coat. Bake for 15 minutes or
until the sweet potato starts to soften. Turn over
and add the broccoli with a little more oil. Bake for
10 minutes.

**2** Add the kale and drizzle with a little more oil, and
season. Bake for 3 minutes until starting to crisp.
**3** To make the dressing, whisk all the ingredients
together with a little water. Divide the vegetables
between two bowls, add the chickpea crunchies
and pour over the dressing. Scatter with
pomegranate seeds and serve.

# Barbecue Tempeh Bowl

 **V** **VE**

NUTRITIONAL INFORMATION PER SERVING 430 Kcals, **Protein** 26.8g, **Carbohydrates** 28.2g
of which sugars 19.3g, **Fat** 20.4g of which saturates 5.6g

SERVES 2   PREPARATION: 15 minutes, plus making the barbecue sauce and 1 hour or overnight marinating
COOKING: 6 minutes

✛200g/7oz tempeh, cut into 2cm/¾in strips, or firm tofu, cut into chunks ✛½ × quantity Fruity Barbecue Sauce
(page 71) ✛1 tbsp coconut oil ✛3 large handfuls of mixed leafy greens, such as baby spinach, watercress,
chopped kale, chicory, rocket/arugula ✛8 cherry tomatoes, cut in half ✛⅓ cucumber, cut in half lengthways, then
cut into slices ✛150g/5½oz/1 small raw beetroot/beet or carrot, grated ✛2 spring onions/scallions, chopped
✛½ avocado, pitted, skinned and sliced ✛2 tbsp pitted black olives, cut in half

**1** Put the tempeh in a shallow dish and pour over
half the barbecue sauce to coat. Transfer to the
refrigerator to marinate for 1 hour or overnight.
**2** Heat the oil in a frying pan over a medium heat.
Add the tempeh and cook on each side for
5–6 minutes until golden and crisp. Remove from

the pan and leave to one side.
**3** Divide the greens between two bowls. Add the
tomatoes, cucumber and beetroot/beet. Scatter
over the spring onions/scallions. Top with the
avocado, olives and fried tempeh. Drizzle over the
remaining barbecue sauce, then serve.

# Massaged-Greens Bowl

**V** NUTRITIONAL INFORMATION PER SERVING 455 Kcals, **Protein** 13.6g,
Carbohydrates 7.3g of which sugars 6.9g, **Fat** 40.2g of which saturates 6.2g

SERVES 2   PREPARATION: 15 minutes   COOKING: 6 minutes

+ 30g/1oz/scant ¼ cup walnuts, roughly broken + ½ tsp garlic powder + ½ tsp onion powder + 1 tsp olive oil
+ 2 eggs + 1 large head of romaine lettuce, cut into large chunks + 2 handfuls of watercress or rocket/arugula
+ 8 mangetout/snow peas, sliced + 1 apple, cored and diced + 2 celery stalks, finely diced + 1 small handful of
flat-leaf parsley leaves  ALMOND DRESSING + ¼ tsp Dijon mustard + 2 tsp apple cider vinegar + 1½ tbsp extra
virgin olive oil or flaxseed oil + 1 tbsp almond or cashew nut butter + sea salt and ground black pepper

**1** Preheat the oven to 180°C/350°F/Gas 4 and
lightly grease a baking sheet. Put the walnuts in a
bowl and stir in the garlic and onion powders, the
oil and a pinch of salt. Spread the walnuts on the
prepared baking sheet. Cook in the oven for
5–6 minutes until the nuts are lightly crisp.
**2** Cook the eggs according to your taste: either
cracked and poached in a frying pan half-filled with
boiling water for 5 minutes; or hard-boiled for

10 minutes, cooled under cold water, then shelled.
**3** To make the dressing, put the ingredients into a
blender, add 3 tbsp water and whiz until smooth.
**4** Put the lettuce, watercress, mangetout/snow
peas, apple and celery in a large bowl. Add half the
dressing and lightly massage into the vegetables.
Divide the vegetables between two bowls, scatter
with parsley, and top with the eggs. Add the walnuts,
drizzle over a little more dressing, then serve.

# Leftovers Sushi Bowl

NUTRITIONAL INFORMATION PER SERVING 348 Kcals, **Protein** 23g,
**Carbohydrates** 20.1g of which sugars 7.6g, **Fat** 17.3g of which saturates 3.2g

SERVES 2   PREPARATION: 15 minutes, plus making the dressing   COOKING: 15 minutes

+ 3 tbsp quinoa, or 80g/2¾oz/½ cup Cauliflower Rice (page 167) + 80g/2¾oz/½ cup shelled frozen edamame
+ 100g/3½oz smoked or leftover poached salmon, thinly sliced + 100g/3½oz/½ daikon or 2 red radishes, sliced
+ ⅓ cucumber, cut lengthways, then sliced + 1 carrot, peeled and grated + ½ avocado, pitted, skinned and sliced
+ 2 tbsp pickled ginger + 1 sheet of nori, crumbled + 1 tbsp sesame seeds + Miso Tahini Orange Dressing (page 125)

**1** Rinse the quinoa well, then put it in a saucepan
and cover with water. Bring to the boil over a
high heat, then reduce the heat and simmer for
15 minutes or until tender. Turn off the heat and
leave to steam for a further 5 minutes. Drain in a
sieve/fine-mesh strainer and leave to cool.

**2** Meanwhile, cook the edamame in boiling water
for 5 minutes. Drain and leave to cool.
**3** Divide the quinoa between two bowls. Put the
salmon, vegetables and avocado on top, then
scatter over the pickled ginger, nori and sesame
seeds. Drizzle with miso dressing and serve.

NUTRITIONAL INFORMATION PER SERVING (based on chicken) 236 Kcals, **Protein** 36.2g, **Carbohydrates** 9.5g of which sugars 4.5g, **Fat** 5.2g of which saturates 1.2g

# Miso Pot Noodle

Here is my very adaptable twist on pot noodles! The base is key for flavour – use miso, kimchi, coconut cream, tahini, tamari or bouillon stock and plenty of spices. Instead of regular noodles, use kelp noodles or spiralized vegetables. You can use leftover cooked vegetables, or add frozen veg to your jar the night before and store it in the refrigerator. Use whatever protein you have – cooked meat, fish or prawns/shrimp, a hard-boiled egg or canned lentils or beans, diced tofu or cooked tempeh. Pack your noodle-pot components in layers to keep the dry and wet ingredients separate, then store the jars in the refrigerator.

Serves 2

Preparation: 10 minutes, plus
  making the kimchi

2 tbsp white miso paste

2 tsp tamari soy sauce

2 tbsp Kimchi (page 68) or 1cm/
  ½in piece of root ginger, peeled
  and grated, and 1 garlic clove,
  crushed

60g/2¼oz/½ cup frozen peas

2 shiitake mushrooms, thinly sliced

1 large handful of baby spinach
  leaves, torn

200g/7oz cooked chicken,
  shredded, or cooked prawns/
  shrimp, or cooked tempeh

2 small courgettes/zucchini,
  spiralized, or 70g/2½oz kelp
  noodles, soaked for 10 minutes
  and drained

1 spring onion/scallion, finely sliced

1 handful of bean sprouts

1 tbsp chopped fresh coriander/
  cilantro leaves

**1** You will need two heatproof containers. Put the miso paste, tamari and kimchi in the base of both containers. Layer the vegetables and chicken and top with the courgette/zucchini noodles, spring onions/scallions, bean sprouts and coriander/cilantro leaves.

**2** Seal the jars and refrigerate until ready to eat. The jars can be packed 1 day ahead and stored in the refrigerator.

**3** When ready to eat, pour over some boiling water and stir well, then allow the noodles to soak for 2 minutes before eating.

## Brain Benefits

Spinach is packed with antioxidants and phytochemicals that help improve blood flow and reduce inflammation – good blood flow is critical to brain function. It also provides B vitamins, folate, vitamin K, zinc and magnesium – all vital nutrients for optimal brain health.

# Garlic Broccoli, Lentil & Tomato Salad

Wonderful served warm, this is a generous salad bursting with goodness. Using cooked lentils makes it a speedy option for a healthy fast lunch, too. If you prefer to cook the lentils yourself, use 100g/3½oz/ ½ cup dried Puy lentils and cook according to the package directions.

Serves 2
Preparation: 15 minutes
Cooking: 8 minutes

1½ heads of broccoli, cut into
  florets
1 tbsp coconut or olive oil
2 garlic cloves, thinly sliced
1 red chilli, deseeded and sliced
1 small red onion, diced
250g/9oz/2½ cups cooked Puy
  lentils
125g/4½oz/¾ cup cherry tomatoes,
  cut in half
1 tbsp balsamic vinegar
1 handful of parsley leaves,
  chopped
sea salt and ground black pepper

**1** Bring a saucepan of lightly salted water to the boil and blanch the broccoli florets for 2–3 minutes until al dente. Drain in a colander, then refresh in cold water to keep the colour. Drain and dry on paper towels.

**2** Heat the oil in a large frying pan and add the garlic, chilli and onion. Cook for 2 minutes. Add the broccoli and mix into the onion mixture, then tip in the lentils and tomatoes, and cook for 2 minutes to heat through. Pour over the vinegar and cook for 1 minute. Season with salt and pepper and scatter over the parsley, then serve.

### Brain Benefits

Eating broccoli can enhance your body's ability to detoxify, thanks to the phytochemical sulforaphane. It also contains selenium, a mineral with antioxidant properties, which supports the production of glutathione – the body's most powerful antioxidant. By protecting fat and lipid cells, selenium improves the health and function of the cellular membranes, including the brain cells.

**P** NUTRITIONAL INFORMATION PER SERVING 153 Kcals, **Protein** 6.7g,
**Carbohydrates** 14.3g of which sugars 13.8g, **Fat** 6.1g of which saturates 0.9g

# Vegetable Ribbons with Puttanesca

Enjoy this gutsy sauce tossed through coloured vegetable noodles for a low-carbohydrate salad. Serve it warm or cold and, for additional protein, toss in some cooked beans, fish or seafood, if you like.

Serves 2

Preparation: 15 minutes

Cooking: 10 minutes, plus
    5 minutes resting

2 courgettes/zucchini, spiralized

1 carrot or beetroot/beet, spiralized

½ cucumber, spiralized

basil leaves, to garnish

FOR THE SAUCE

3 anchovy fillets in oil, drained and
    finely chopped

2 garlic cloves, chopped

a pinch of dried chilli/hot pepper
    flakes

400g/14oz can plum tomatoes

80g/2¾oz/¾ cup pitted black
    olives, cut in half

1 handful of basil leaves, roughly
    chopped or torn

1 tbsp capers, drained and rinsed

8 cherry tomatoes, cut in half

2 tsp balsamic or apple cider
    vinegar

ground black pepper

**1** Put all the ingredients for the sauce in a large saucepan over a medium heat and bring to the boil, then reduce the heat and simmer, covered, for 10 minutes, breaking up the tomatoes occasionally with a wooden spoon.

**2** Add the vegetables to the pan and toss into the sauce to coat thoroughly. Turn off the heat and allow the vegetables to rest in the sauce for 5 minutes before serving so that they soften slightly. Serve warm or leave to cool and serve cold, garnished with basil.

**Brain Benefits**

Beetroot/beet and beetroot juice contain high concentrations of nitrates, which are converted into nitrites and nitric oxide in the stomach in the body. These help increase blood flow and oxygen to the brain, which can help to improve focus, concentration and cognitive function.

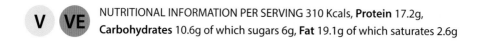

NUTRITIONAL INFORMATION PER SERVING 310 Kcals, **Protein** 17.2g,
**Carbohydrates** 10.6g of which sugars 6g, **Fat** 19.1g of which saturates 2.6g

# Lemon & Tahini Wilted Kale & Nori Salad

**Calcium-rich tahini lends a rich flavour to this creamy and tangy dairy-free salad. By massaging the dressing into the kale leaves, you will soften their texture so that they take on a wilted appearance.**

Serves 2
Preparation: 15 minutes
Cooking: 3 minutes

2 tbsp mixed seeds
8 asparagus spears
300g/10½oz kale, chopped
2 sheets of nori, torn
8 cherry tomatoes, cut in half
¼ cucumber, cut in half lengthways
    and sliced

**FOR THE TAHINI LEMON DRESSING**
½ tsp onion powder
½ tsp garlic salt
1 tsp tamari soy sauce
½ tsp apple cider vinegar
½ tsp ground cumin
½ red pepper/bell pepper,
    deseeded and chopped
zest and juice of ½ lemon
2 tbsp tahini
2 tbsp nutritional yeast flakes

**1** Put the seeds in a small saucepan and toast them over a medium-high heat for 30 seconds or until evenly toasted, shaking the pan frequently. Tip out of the pan onto a plate.

**2** Bring a saucepan of water to the boil and blanch the asparagus for 2–3 minutes until al dente, then drain in a colander. Leave to cool, then cut into 3cm/1¼in pieces.

**3** To make the dressing, put all the ingredients into a blender or food processor and add 2 tablespoons water. Whiz until smooth, adding more water if needed to make a thick and creamy dressing.

**4** Put the kale in a large bowl and pour over the dressing. With your hands, massage the dressing into the kale so that it softens and wilts.

**5** Mix in the nori, asparagus, tomatoes and cucumber. Scatter over the toasted seeds and serve.

### Brain Benefits

Kale and asparagus are packed with B vitamins, folate and magnesium, which are essential for the production of neurotransmitters. The seeds contain healthy fats, zinc and vitamin E, which all have an important role to play in cognitive function.

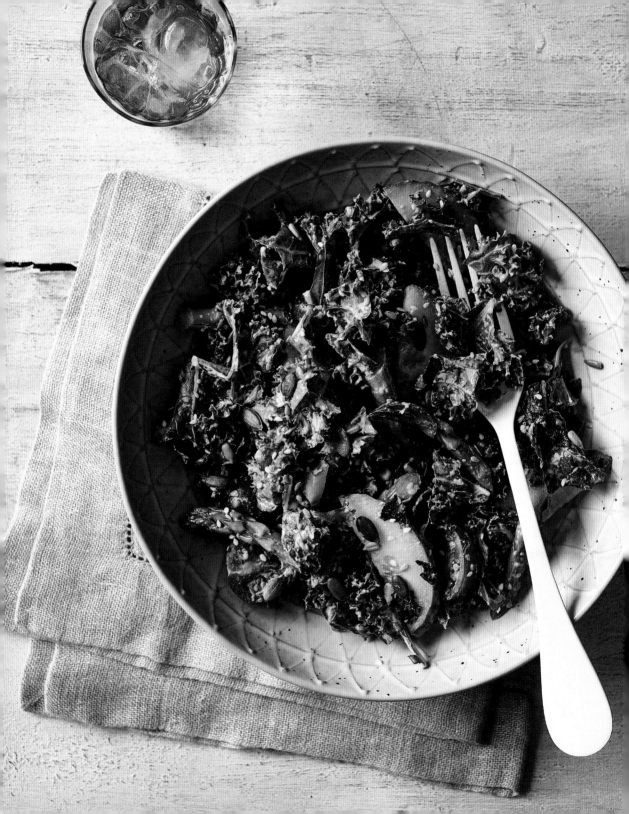

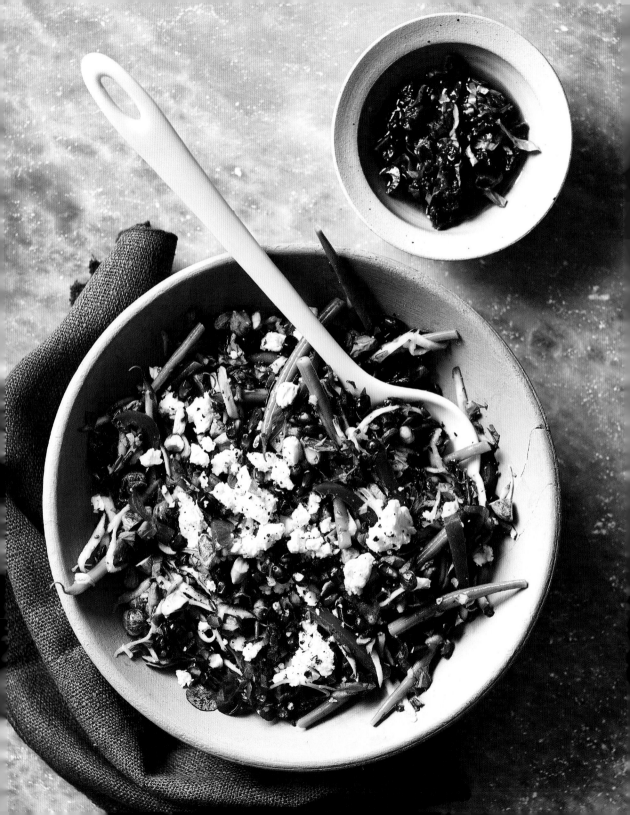

**V** NUTRITIONAL INFORMATION PER SERVING (with 1 tbsp dressing) 471 Kcals, **Protein** 13.3g, **Carbohydrates** 38.7g of which sugars 7.2g, **Fat** 27.6g of which saturates 5.5g

# Mediterranean Red Rice Salad with Pomegranate & Feta

Sweet pomegranate complements the sharpness of feta in this mixed salad full of fresh flavours and crunch. Store the leftover dressing in the fridge and use to drizzle over salads or steamed vegetables.

Serves 2
Preparation: 15 minutes
Cooking: 20–30 minutes

80g/2¾oz/½ cup red rice
100g/3½oz fine green beans
50g/1¾oz/½ cup pistachio nuts
2 tsp olive oil
finely grated zest of 1 lemon
1 tbsp capers, drained and rinsed
½ red pepper/bell pepper,
    deseeded and cut into thin
    matchsticks
1 courgette/zucchini, coarsely
    grated
1 handful of watercress, chopped
2 tbsp chopped parsley leaves
30g/1oz feta cheese, crumbled
2 tbsp fresh pomegranate seeds

FOR THE DRESSING
6 sun-dried tomatoes in oil, drained
    and chopped
4 pitted black olives, finely chopped
1 tbsp finely chopped basil leaves
2 tbsp red wine or balsamic vinegar
2 tbsp extra virgin olive oil

**1** Put the rice in a saucepan and add double the volume of water. Bring to the boil, then simmer for 20–30 minutes or until tender, or according to the package directions. Drain and leave to one side.

**2** To make the dressing, put all the ingredients in a bowl and whisk them together. Bring a saucepan of water to the boil and blanch the green beans for 2–3 minutes until al dente. Drain in a colander.

**3** Put the nuts in a frying pan and toast them over a medium heat for 1–2 minutes or until just golden, shaking the pan frequently. Tip out of the pan onto a plate.

**4** Add the olive oil to the frying pan, then add the lemon zest, capers, red pepper/bell pepper and courgette/zucchini. Stir-fry for 2 minutes or until hot and just beginning to turn golden. Add the rice, green beans, watercress and parsley, and continue to stir-fry for 2 minutes, or until heated through. Drizzle over a little of the dressing and scatter the toasted nuts, feta cheese and pomegranate seeds over the top, then serve.

### Brain Benefits

Red rice is rich in anthocyanidins, which are potent antioxidants (the same found in berries) that protect the body and brain. It also provides a good source of iron, zinc and manganese, plus B vitamins to support brain function and energy production.

# Dressings

A good salad dressing can transform your leaves and can completely change the way you think about greens. They are an excellent way of spicing up and experimenting with a whole range of vegetables, as well as including even more beneficial ingredients. These dressing recipes are perfect for incorporating plenty of cleansing and anti-inflammatory ingredients as well as healthy fats – all essential for a healthy brain.

Use the dressings over raw or cooked vegetables, beans or gluten-free grains. You can experiment with different oils, citrus flavours and herbs to find your own favourites.

*These dressings are perfect for incorporating plenty of cleansing and anti-inflammatory ingredients.*

## Super-Green Herb Dressing

 NUTRITIONAL INFORMATION PER 1 TBSP 15 Kcals, **Protein** 0.6g, **Carbohydrates** 0.8g of which sugars 0.5g, **Fat** 1g of which saturates 0.7g

MAKES about 300ml/10½fl oz/scant 1⅓ cups  PREPARATION: 5 minutes

✢1 garlic clove, crushed  ✢200g/7oz/1 cup Greek yogurt or coconut yogurt, or use half and half with mayonnaise ✢2 tbsp apple cider vinegar  ✢juice of ½ lemon  ✢2 tbsp extra virgin olive oil, or avocado oil, or a combination of macadamia nut oil with MCT oil  ✢1 large handful of basil leaves  ✢1 large handful of parsley leaves  ✢1 handful of tarragon leaves  ✢1 handful of chives  ✢1 tsp sea salt  ✢1 tsp xylitol or erythritol, or to taste

**1** Put all the ingredients into a blender or food processor and whiz until smooth. Store in an airtight container in the refrigerator for up to 1 week or freeze for up to 3 months.

**Brain Benefits**
Using yogurt is a perfect way of including beneficial bacteria for overall digestive health, while the fresh herbs provide plenty of antioxidant and anti-inflammatory benefits.

# Miso Tahini Orange Dressing

 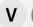 NUTRITIONAL INFORMATION PER 1 TBSP 41 Kcals, **Protein** 1.4g, **Carbohydrates** 0.8g of which sugars 0.3g, **Fat** 3.4g of which saturates 0.5g

MAKES about 115ml/3¾fl oz/scant ½ cup PREPARATION: 5 minutes

✢2 tbsp tahini ✢1 tbsp hot water ✢1 tbsp white miso paste ✢2 tbsp orange juice ✢1 tsp sesame oil ✢2 tsp apple cider vinegar ✢½ garlic clove, crushed

1 Put all the ingredients into a blender or food processor and whiz until smooth and creamy. Store in an airtight container in the refrigerator for up to 1 week.

**Brain Benefits**
Miso is a delicious fermented paste and an easy way to add additional probiotics. This dressing can also be used to replace the miso gravy in the Mushroom Buddha Bowl on page 176.

---

# Mint & Caper Dressing

 NUTRITIONAL INFORMATION PER 1 TBSP 97 Kcals, **Protein** 0.2g, **Carbohydrates** 0.1g of which sugars 0.1g, **Fat** 10.6g of which saturates 1.5g

MAKES about 300ml/10½fl oz/scant 1⅓ cups PREPARATION: 5 minutes

✢4 tbsp finely chopped basil leaves ✢3 tbsp finely chopped parsley leaves ✢3 tbsp finely chopped mint leaves ✢1 tbsp capers, rinsed, drained and roughly chopped ✢1 tsp Dijon mustard ✢4 anchovy fillets in oil, drained and roughly chopped ✢2 tbsp lemon juice, apple cider vinegar or Homemade Kombucha (page 65) ✢a pinch of garlic salt ✢200ml/7fl oz/scant 1 cup extra virgin olive oil

1 Put all the ingredients in a bowl and whisk together. Store in an airtight container in the refrigerator for up to 4 days.

**Brain Benefits**
Capers are one of the highest plant sources of the flavonoid antioxidants rutin and quercetin. Quercetin is particularly known for its anti-inflammatory benefits, and rutin for its circulatory qualities.

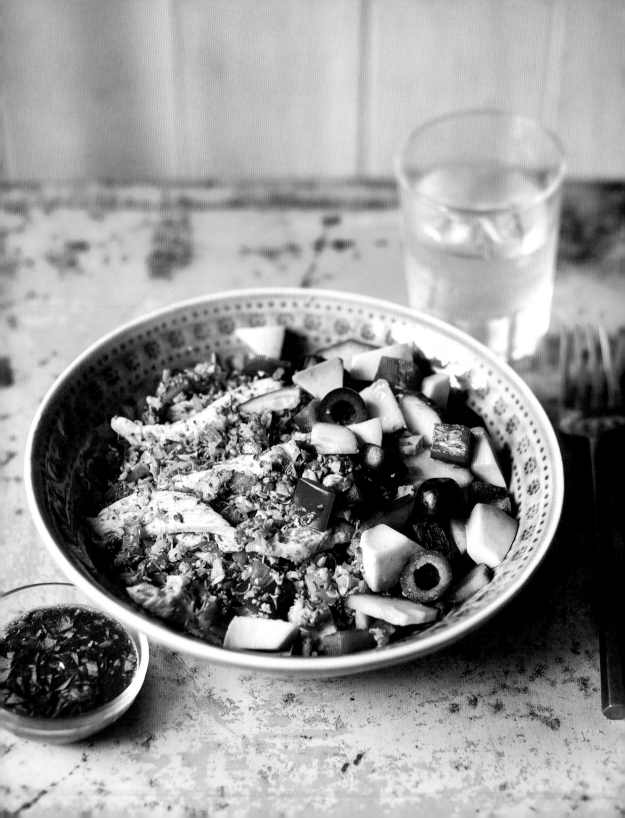

**P** NUTRITIONAL INFORMATION PER SERVING (with 1 tbsp dressing) 449 Kcals, **Protein** 40.8g, **Carbohydrates** 11.1g of which sugars 7.7g, **Fat** 24.2g of which saturates 6g

# Chicken Burrito Bowl

A lovely one-bowl dish full of fresh flavours, this salad is a perfect way to use up leftover meat and veggies. The toasted garlic dressing is full of punchy flavours and is just as delicious poured over cooked vegetables or pulses. Add some salad greens and coriander/cilantro to the bowl for extra freshness.

Serves 2
Preparation: 20 minutes
Cooking: 5 minutes

4 garlic cloves, peeled and left
    whole
½ tsp Dijon mustard
1 tbsp chopped parsley leaves
2 tbsp balsamic vinegar
4 tbsp extra virgin olive oil
1 head of broccoli, cut into florets
1 tbsp coconut oil
1 small onion, chopped
1 tsp smoked paprika
¼ tsp cayenne pepper or taco
    seasoning
200g/7oz cooked chicken, shredded
½ cucumber, cut in half and thinly
    sliced
½ red pepper/bell pepper,
    deseeded and diced
30g/1oz/⅓ cup pitted black olives,
    cut in half
½ avocado, pitted, skinned and
    diced

**1** Put the garlic cloves in a non-stick frying pan and toast for 1 minute or until the garlic has turned golden. Leave to cool, then crush the garlic. Put in a screwtop jar and add the mustard, parsley, vinegar and oil, then shake to mix thoroughly. (This dressing can be stored in the refrigerator for up to 3 days.)

**2** Put the broccoli in a food processor, or electric chopper, and pulse gently to form rice-like grains. Leave to one side.

**3** Heat half the coconut oil in a frying pan over a medium heat. Add the onion and cook gently for 2 minutes or until softened. Tip in the broccoli and spices, and stir to coat in the oil. Cover and steam-fry for 2 minutes to soften the broccoli slightly. Add the cooked chicken and mix well.

**4** Put the cucumber in a bowl and add the red pepper/bell pepper, olives and avocado. Mix well. Divide the broccoli rice between two bowls. Divide the cucumber mixture between the bowls. Drizzle over a little of the dressing and serve.

**Brain Benefits**

Diets high in extra virgin olive oil, including Mediterranean diets, are known for their lower incidence of cognitive decline and cardiovascular disease. Extra virgin olive oil is rich in monounsaturated fat and phenolics, which can help to reduce oxidative damage and lower inflammation.

**P** NUTRITIONAL INFORMATION PER SERVING 142 Kcals, **Protein** 19.1g, **Carbohydrates** 11.6g of which sugars 6.9g, **Fat** 1.3g of which saturates 0.2g

# Vietnamese Prawn Salad

This wonderful sweet-and-sour salad has classic Thai flavours. It uses raw prawns/shrimp but you could substitute ready-cooked prawns if you prefer and just add them to the vegetables. It's a light protein-packed dish that is perfect for intermittent-fasting days.

Serves 2

Preparation: 15 minutes

Cooking: 5 minutes

200g/7oz large raw prawns/shrimp, peeled

1 carrot, cut into thin matchsticks

½ red pepper/bell pepper, deseeded and cut into thin matchsticks

½ cucumber, deseeded and thinly sliced or spiralized

½ red onion, thinly sliced

½ red chilli, deseeded and chopped

1 handful of fresh mint leaves

1 handful of fresh coriander/cilantro leaves

FOR THE THAI DRESSING

4 tbsp lime juice

2 tsp xylitol or erythritol

1 tbsp Thai fish sauce

½ garlic clove, crushed

5mm/¼in piece of root ginger, peeled and grated

1 lemongrass stalk, lower part only, sliced

**1** To make the dressing, put all the ingredients in a blender or mini food processor and whiz until combined. Leave to one side.

**2** Make a shallow cut down the centre of the curved back of each prawn/shrimp. Pull out the black vein with a cocktail stick/toothpick or your fingers, then rinse the prawn thoroughly.

**3** Bring a saucepan of water to the boil, then reduce the heat to a simmer. Add the prawns and simmer for 3 minutes or until they turn pink. Drain in a colander, and rinse.

**4** Put all the vegetables in a large bowl and add the chilli, herbs and prawns, then toss together well. When ready to serve, pour over the dressing and toss well, then serve.

## Brain Benefits

Red peppers/bell peppers are one of the best sources of lycopene, a potent antioxidant known to help protect the body from damage by free-radicals. Red peppers also contain pyridoxine (vitamin B6), which plays an important role in brain function, plus the antioxidant vitamins C and A.

**P** NUTRITIONAL INFORMATION PER SERVING 396 Kcals, **Protein** 32.3g, **Carbohydrates** 3.8g of which sugars 3.1g, **Fat** 27g of which saturates 5g

# Moroccan-Spiced Salmon Niçoise

Fresh and crunchy, this salad contains nourishing omega-3 fats and cleansing greens. Ras el hanout adds a North African flavour, for a wonderfully warming, aromatic version of the traditional Niçoise salad.

Serves 2
Preparation: 15 minutes
Cooking: 12–15 minutes

1 tbsp capers, drained, rinsed and
   chopped
½ anchovy in oil, rinsed and finely
   chopped
2 tbsp red wine vinegar
1½ tsp ras el hanout
2 tbsp extra virgin olive oil
2 tbsp chopped fresh herbs, such as
   parsley, basil
2 tsp olive oil
zest of ½ lemon
1 tsp yacon syrup or other liquid
   sweetener
2 boneless salmon fillets with skin,
   120g/4¼oz each
100g/3½oz green beans
1 Little Gem/mini romaine lettuce,
   leaves separated
1 large handful of rocket/arugula,
   watercress or dandelion greens
8 cherry tomatoes, cut in half
30g/1oz/⅓ cup pitted black olives,
   cut in half
1 hard-boiled egg, cut into quarters
sea salt and ground black pepper

**1** Put the capers in a small bowl and add the anchovy, vinegar, ½ teaspoon of the ras el hanout, the extra virgin olive oil and herbs. Whisk together, then season with salt and pepper. (This dressing can be stored in the refrigerator for up to 3 days.)

**2** Preheat the oven to 200°C/400°F/Gas 6. Put the olive oil in a bowl and add the lemon zest, the remaining ras el hanout and the yacon syrup, then spread this mixture over the salmon fillets. Season with salt and pepper and put in a roasting pan. Cook in the oven for 12–15 minutes until the salmon is cooked through. Remove from the oven and leave to cool. Flake into large chunks.

**3** Meanwhile, bring a saucepan of water to the boil and blanch the beans for 2–3 minutes until just soft. Drain in a colander and refresh in cold water to keep the colour. Drain well.

**4** Divide the lettuce and rocket/arugula between the plates, top with the beans, tomatoes and olives, then scatter over the flaked salmon and add the egg quarters. Drizzle with the dressing and serve.

### Brain Benefits

Salmon, particularly wild salmon, is one of the best protein sources for brain health. It contains high levels of omega-3 fats and docosahexaenoic acid (DHA) which accounts for more than two-thirds of the brain's fatty acids. It also provides protective vitamins A and C. Bitter greens support digestive health and provide prebiotic fibre to support a diverse range of beneficial bacteria in the gut.

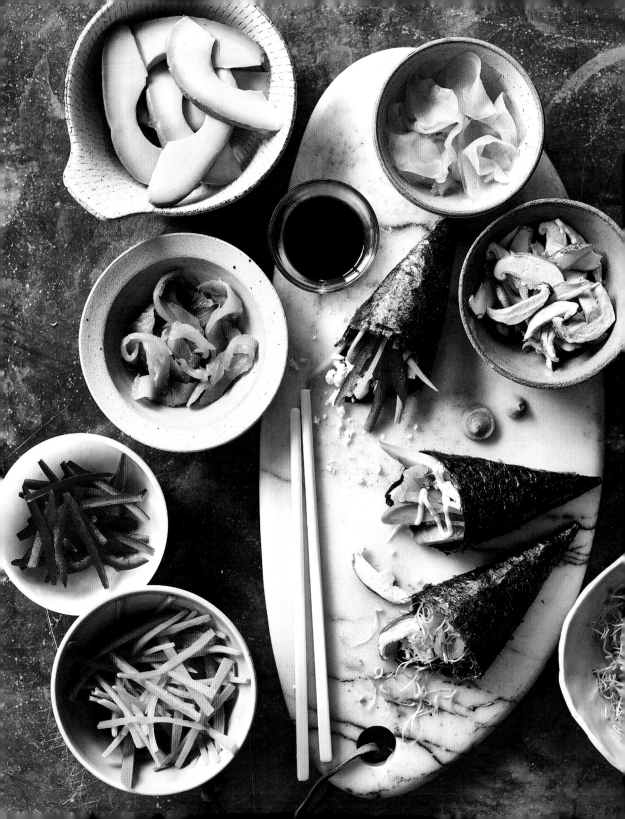

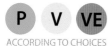

NUTRITIONAL INFORMATION PER SERVING 355 Kcals, **Protein** 8.3g, **Carbohydrates** 5.5g of which sugars 3.9g, **Fat** 32.3g of which saturates 3.5g

# Speedy Nori Hand Rolls with Spicy Mayo

Rather than using traditional refined white rice for nori rolls, these low-carb options use cauliflower rice as a filling with smoked salmon and colourful veggies. You can change the fillings: instead of salmon you could use chopped cooked prawns/shrimp, or sprouted beans and tofu for a veggie option.

Serves 2

Preparation: 20 minutes, plus
    making the mayonnaise

150g/5½oz cauliflower, broken into
    florets
30g/1oz macadamia nuts or cashew
    nuts
a pinch of sea salt
1 tsp umeboshi vinegar or apple
    cider vinegar
1 tsp white miso paste
3 tbsp Blender Mayonnaise
    (page 70)
½–1 tsp wasabi paste, to taste
a pinch of xylitol or erythritol
4 nori sheets
pickled ginger and tamari, to serve

FOR THE FILLING
Choose your favourites from:
    strips of smoked salmon
    enoki mushrooms or thin strips
        of shiitake mushrooms
    alfalfa sprouts
    thin matchsticks of carrots
        or deseeded red pepper/
        bell pepper
    thin slices of avocado

**1** Put the cauliflower into a food processor, or electric chopper, and add the nuts and salt, then pulse until the mixture looks like couscous. Add the vinegar and miso, and whiz again to combine. Leave to one side.

**2** Mix the mayonnaise with the wasabi and xylitol. Cut each nori sheet in half. Lay a half-nori sheet, shiny-side down, on a large board. Using moistened hands, put a ping-pong ball-size amount of the cauliflower rice on the right side of the nori sheet, then flatten it down slightly to form a rectangle – this should cover about one-third of the sheet.

**3** Smear a small amount of the mayonnaise diagonally across the rice. Put your chosen filling ingredients diagonally on top of the rice so that they point towards the bottom-right corner of the nori. Fold the top-right corner of the nori over the rice and filling ingredients. Pick the hand roll up and wrap the left side of the nori tightly around the rice and fillings to form a cone shape, leaving a small flap. Moisten the flap of nori with water and seal the cone. Repeat with the other 3 rolls.

**4** Leave the rolls for 1–2 minutes before eating to let the rice and fillings soften the nori. Serve with pickled ginger, tamari and the remaining wasabi mayonnaise.

## Brain Benefits

This dish is packed with brain-healthy fats thanks to the addition of the homemade mayo, with iodine to support cognitive function and cauliflower to aid detoxification.

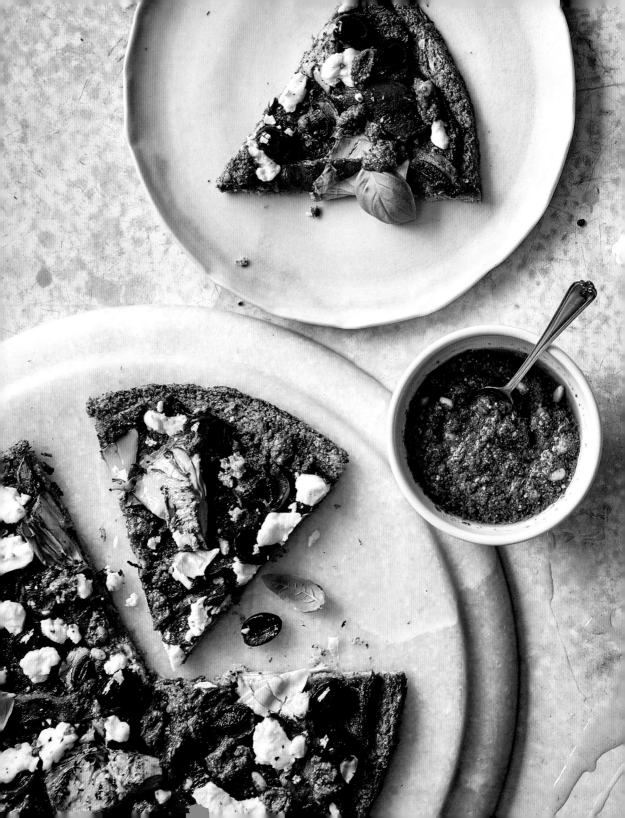

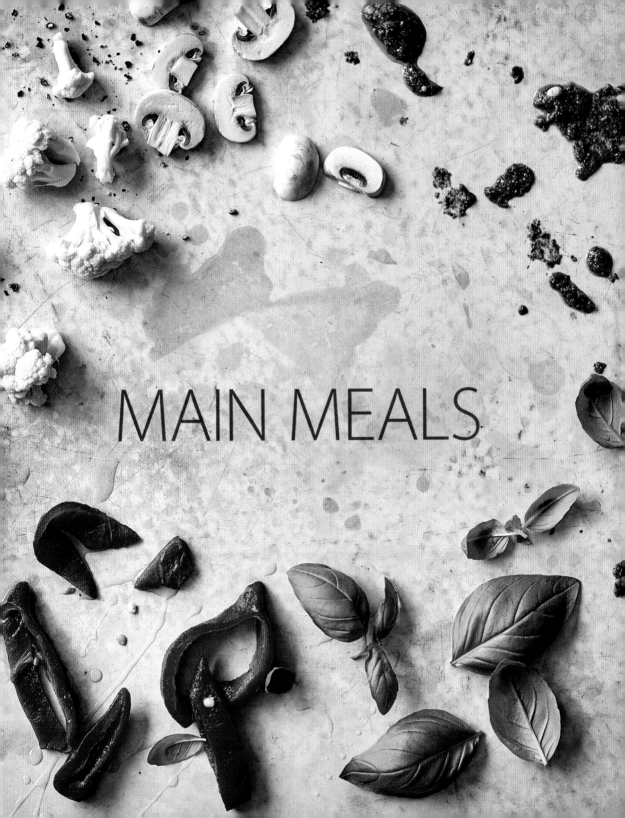

# MAIN MEALS

**P** NUTRITIONAL INFORMATION PER SERVING 550 Kcals, **Protein** 31.7g, **Carbohydrates** 21.7g of which sugars 13g, **Fat** 36.2g of which saturates 12.3g

# Meatballs with Butternut Squash Pasta

Using butternut squash as pasta gives this dish plenty of colour; it's more nourishing and tastes great combined with crunchy pine nuts. You could also use carrots or sweet potato.

Serves 2
Preparation: 20 minutes, plus 30
    minutes chilling
Cooking: 25 minutes

30g/1oz/¼ cup pine nuts
250g/9oz/scant 1¼ cups lean
    minced/ground lamb
2 sun-dried tomatoes in oil, drained
    and finely chopped
2 garlic cloves, crushed
8 sage leaves, finely chopped
1 egg yolk
1 tbsp arrowroot powder or
    cornflour/cornstarch
400g/14oz can chopped tomatoes
½ red onion, finely chopped
2 tsp balsamic vinegar
2 tsp coconut oil
½ butternut squash, peeled,
    deseeded and spiralized
1 tsp olive oil
1 handful of pitted black olives, cut
    in half
sea salt and ground black pepper

**1** Put the pine nuts in a small saucepan and toast them over a medium-high heat for 1–2 minutes or until evenly toasted, shaking the pan frequently. Tip out of the pan onto a plate and leave to one side.

**2** Put the lamb in a large bowl and add the sun-dried tomatoes, 1 crushed garlic clove, 4 sage leaves, the egg yolk and arrowroot. Season with salt and pepper, and mix together with your hands. Roll the mixture into golf-ball-size portions, then put them in the refrigerator to chill for 30 minutes or until ready to cook.

**3** Put the chopped tomatoes in a small pan over a medium-high heat and add the onion and vinegar. Season and bring to the boil, then reduce the heat and simmer for 10 minutes to thicken slightly.

**4** Heat the coconut oil in a large frying pan and fry the meatballs for 3–4 minutes until golden on one side. Turn them and cook for a further 3–4 minutes until cooked through. Add the tomato sauce and return to the boil, then reduce the heat, cover and simmer for 2 minutes.

**5** Meanwhile, put the butternut squash in a separate frying pan and add the olive oil, the remaining garlic and sage, the toasted pine nuts and olives, then season. Cover the pan and cook for 1–2 minutes until the squash is just tender. Serve with the meatballs and tomato sauce.

### Brain Benefits
Pine nuts contain a wide range of antioxidants: vitamins A, B, C, D and E, and lutein. These are crucial to brain health, helping to combat free-radicals. Butternut squash adds nourishment in the form of protective antioxidants, including carotenoids and fibre for a healthy gut.

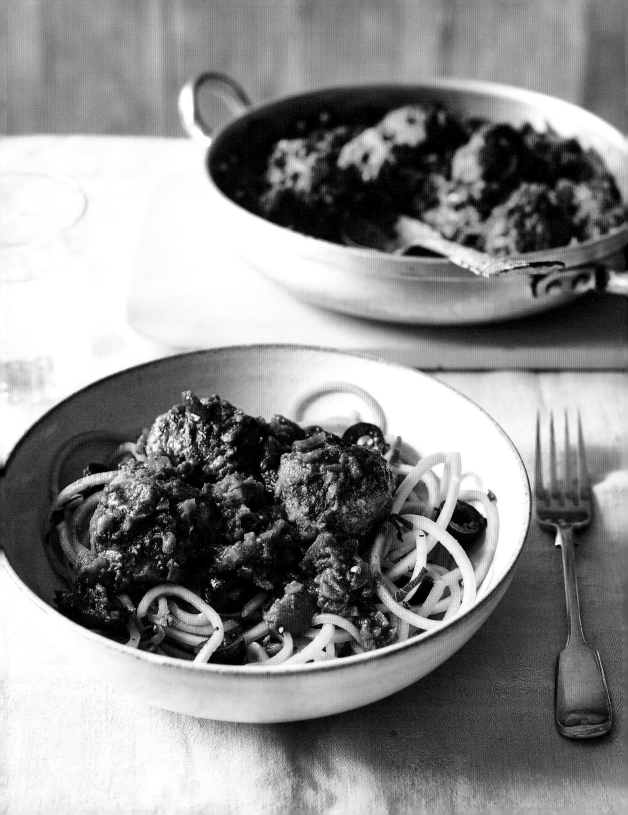

**P** NUTRITIONAL INFORMATION PER SERVING 344 Kcals, **Protein** 26.6g, **Carbohydrates** 1.9g of which sugars 1.2g, **Fat** 25.5g of which saturates 9.2g

# Thai-Spiced Burgers

Burgers can be surprisingly healthy when you ditch the bun. These are quick and simple to make and packed with flavour, making use of bought Thai red curry paste and fresh herbs to give them a kick. As an alternative to serving them on the mushrooms, you can serve them in lettuce leaves, if you prefer.

Serves 2

Preparation: 15 minutes, plus
   30 minutes chilling

Cooking: 20–25 minutes

250g/9oz/scant 1¼ cups lean
   minced/ground lamb or turkey
1 shallot, finely grated
1 garlic clove, crushed
4 sun-dried tomatoes in oil, drained
   and finely chopped
1 tbsp chopped coriander/cilantro
   leaves
1 egg yolk
2 tsp Thai red curry paste
coconut oil, for greasing
2 portobello mushrooms
olive oil, for drizzling
sea salt and ground black pepper
slices of tomato and red onion,
   to serve

1 Put the mince in a large bowl and add the shallot, garlic, sun-dried tomatoes, coriander/cilantro, egg yolk and curry paste. Use your hands to mix everything together well. Season with salt and pepper.

2 Divide and shape the mixture into 2 large burgers or 4 smaller patties. Put on a plate and cover, then chill for 30 minutes.

3 Preheat the oven to 200°C/400°F/Gas 6 and lightly grease a baking sheet. Arrange the burgers on the prepared baking sheet and cook in the oven for 20–25 minutes until they are cooked through, turning once halfway through.

4 Meanwhile, put the mushrooms on a baking sheet and drizzle with the olive oil. Cook in the oven for 5 minutes or until soft. Serve the burgers on the mushrooms and top with slices of tomato and onion.

### Brain Benefits

High in fibre, portobello mushrooms are also an excellent source of copper, which your body needs to produce red blood cells and carry oxygen through your body and brain. They also contain three important B vitamins: riboflavin for maintaining healthy red blood cells to keep the body oxygenated; niacin for skin health and healthy digestive and nervous systems; and pantothenic acid, which aids the production of energy.

NUTRITIONAL INFORMATION PER SERVING 524 Kcals, **Protein** 45.5g, **Carbohydrates** 20.4g of which sugars 17.1 g, **Fat** 26.2g of which saturates 8.2g

# Satay Beef Skewers with Pineapple

**Light and fruity, this dish is flavoured with the nuttiness and creaminess of the peanut sauce contrasted with sweetness from the pineapple.**

Serves 2

Preparation: 15 minutes, plus
chilling and 30 minutes or
overnight marinating

Cooking: 12 minutes

60g/2¼oz/¼ cup peanut butter or
almond nut butter

4 tbsp canned full-fat coconut milk

juice of 1 lime

½ tsp ground cumin

250g/9oz beef sirloin steak, trimmed
of hard fat and cut into thin strips

2 tbsp tamari soy sauce

2 tsp rice malt syrup or yacon syrup

1cm/½in piece of root ginger,
peeled and grated

150g/5½oz fresh pineapple, or
canned pineapple in natural
juice, cut into chunks

2 tsp coconut oil or olive oil

1 garlic clove, crushed

200g/7oz purple sprouting broccoli

1 head of pak choi/bok choy, cut in
half lengthways

chopped mint and coriander/
cilantro leaves, to garnish

lime wedges, to serve

**1** To make the sauce, put the peanut butter in a small saucepan and add the milk, lime juice and cumin. Cook over a low heat, stirring until everything is combined. Tip into a small bowl and leave to cool, then chill in the refrigerator. (You can make this 1–2 days in advance.)

**2** Put the beef in a shallow dish. Put the tamari in a small bowl, add the rice malt syrup and half the ginger, then mix together. Pour this over the beef and leave to marinate for 30 minutes or preferably overnight.

**3** Take four skewers; if using wooden skewers, soak for 30 minutes in water. Thread the pineapple and beef onto the skewers. Reserve the marinade. Heat the grill/broiler to high and put a foil-lined baking sheet beneath the grill/broiling rack. Put the skewers on the rack. Grill/broil the skewers for 3–5 minutes on each side or until cooked to your liking. Brush with some of the reserved marinade during cooking.

**4** Meanwhile, heat the oil in a wok or large saucepan, add the garlic and remaining ginger, and stir-fry for 1 minute. Add the broccoli and a splash of water. Cover and steam-fry for 3 minutes or until just tender. Add the pak choi/bok choy, and cover and cook for 2 minutes or until just soft. Serve the skewers with the greens and sauce, garnished with the herbs and accompanied with lime wedges.

## Brain Benefits

Pineapple is a natural aid for digestion, because it is rich in a natural digestive enzyme known as bromelain, which is also known for its anti-inflammatory properties.

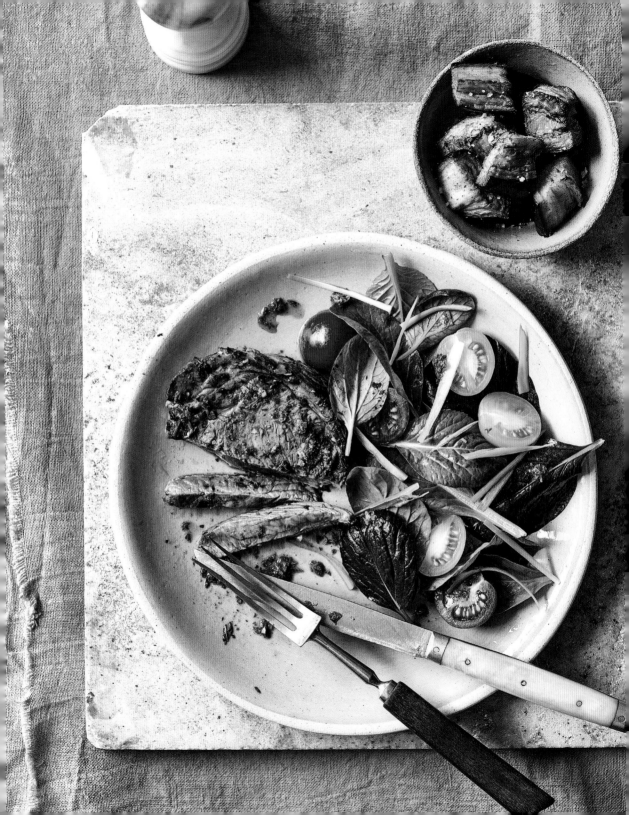

**P** NUTRITIONAL INFORMATION PER SERVING (with 1 tbsp dressing) 315 Kcals, **Protein** 25.8g, **Carbohydrates** 2.9g of which sugars 2.7g, **Fat** 21.6g of which saturates 5.9g

# Grilled Lamb with Aubergine & Minty Chimichurri

In this twist on the traditional spicy chimichurri dressing, an abundance of fresh herbs adds to the overall flavour, and it also has the plus of increasing the health benefits too. Any leftover dressing is delicious drizzled over meat and fish dishes and will keep in the fridge for up to 1 week.

**Serves 2**

**Preparation: 15 minutes, plus 2 hours or overnight marinating**

**Cooking: 20 minutes**

2 lean lamb fillet steaks, 120g/4¼oz each

1 small aubergine/eggplant, cut into chunks

1 tbsp olive oil

1 handful of salad leaves/greens

6 cherry tomatoes, cut in half

1 spring onion/scallion, cut into thin matchsticks

**FOR THE CHIMICHURRI**

1 handful of fresh mint leaves

a small bunch of parsley leaves

1 garlic clove, crushed

¼ tsp smoked paprika

½ tsp ground cumin

1 tbsp lemon juice

5 tbsp extra virgin olive oil

2 tbsp sherry vinegar, or red wine vinegar

sea salt and ground black pepper

**1** To make the chimichurri, put all the ingredients into a blender and whiz to form a chunky sauce. Put the lamb fillets in a shallow container. Spoon half the dressing over and coat the lamb thoroughly. Cover and put in the refrigerator for 2 hours or overnight, if possible.

**2** Preheat the oven to 190°C/375°F/Gas 5. Put the aubergine/eggplant in a roasting pan. Drizzle with the olive oil and season with salt and pepper. Bake for 20 minutes or until the aubergine is soft and lightly golden, stirring occasionally. Remove from the oven and leave to one side.

**3** Meanwhile, heat a griddle/grill pan until hot. Season the lamb with pepper, then pan-fry for 4–5 minutes on each side or until cooked to your liking. Allow the lamb to rest for 5 minutes. Slice thinly.

**4** Serve the lamb with the salad leaves/greens, the aubergine and tomatoes, sprinkled with spring onion/scallion, and drizzled with a little of the dressing.

**Brain Benefits**

Lamb is a rich source of high-quality protein, essential for neurotransmitter production. It is also an outstanding source of many vitamins and minerals, including iron, zinc and vitamin B12. Lamb is also a good source of taurine, a potent neuro-protective amino acid that might also improve sleep patterns and cognitive function.

NUTRITIONAL INFORMATION PER SERVING 193 Kcals, **Protein** 27g,
**Carbohydrates** 7.1g of which sugars 6g, **Fat** 5.6g of which saturates 4.3g

# San Choy Bau

Traditionally made with pork, this version is based on lean turkey to create a tryptophan-rich recipe. The dish is high in protein, and the aromatic spices and herbs are anti-inflammatory. It's also a superb low-carb meal. Sprinkle over some sesame seeds and chopped spring onion/scallion as well, if you like.

Serves 2
Preparation: 15 minutes
Cooking: 9 minutes

1 tbsp coconut oil
1 garlic clove, crushed
5mm/¼in piece of root ginger,
    peeled and grated
½ red onion, finely chopped
½ red chilli, deseeded and chopped
200g/7oz/scant 1 cup lean minced/
    ground turkey
4 shiitake mushrooms, chopped
½ red pepper/bell pepper,
    deseeded and chopped
30g/1oz canned bamboo shoots,
    cut into thin strips
4 canned water chestnuts, chopped
1 tbsp tamari soy sauce
1 tsp fish sauce
2 tbsp mirin
a pinch of Chinese five-spice
    powder
1 tbsp sweet chilli sauce
1 tbsp coriander/cilantro leaves,
    chopped
2 Little Gem/mini romaine lettuces,
    leaves separated, to serve

**1** Heat the oil in a large frying pan over a medium heat. Add the garlic, ginger, onion and chilli, and cook briefly for 1 minute.

**2** Add the turkey, mushrooms, red pepper/bell pepper, bamboo shoots and water chestnuts, and stir-fry for 5 minutes or until the turkey is cooked through.

**3** Add the remaining ingredients except the lettuce. Stir-fry for 2–3 minutes to heat through and soften. Spoon the turkey mixture into the lettuce leaves to serve.

### Brain Benefits

Turkey provides easily absorbable iron, plus zinc and B vitamins for good brain function, and tryptophan to support serotonin production, which can help to boost the mood.

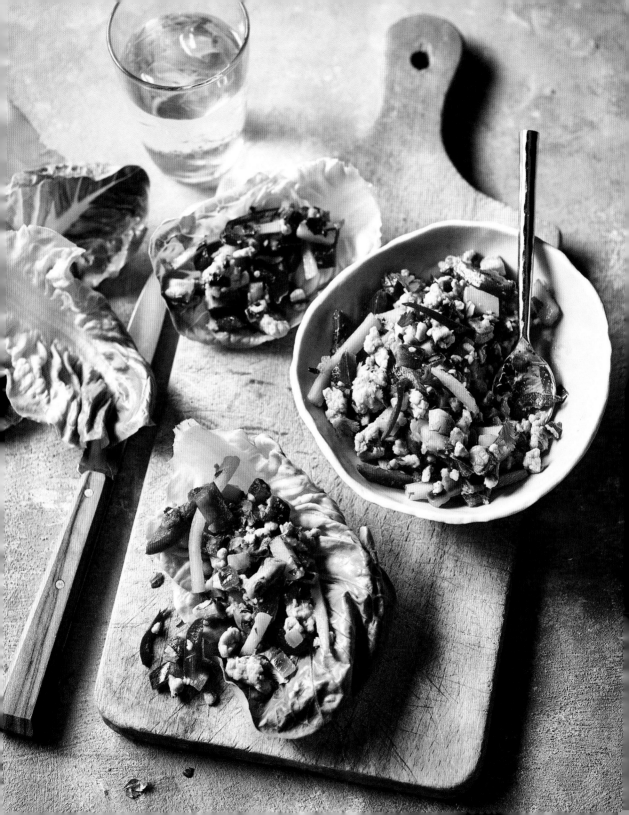

# Crispy Chicken Bites with Avocado Mayo

**Forget fried chicken, these crispy bites are not only much tastier but they are also incredibly simple to prepare. You could make up a large batch of these, freeze them and use from frozen.**

Serves 2

Preparation: 20 minutes, plus
    making the mayonnaise

Cooking: 25 minutes

olive oil, for greasing

1 egg

1 tbsp sriracha hot sauce

80g/2¾oz/½ cup dried red lentils

60g/2¼oz/½ cup almond flour

½ tsp garlic salt

½ tsp smoked paprika

½ tsp onion powder

200g/7oz skinless chicken breasts,
    cut into bite-size pieces

½ small ripe avocado, pitted,
    skinned and chopped

½ garlic clove, crushed

1 tbsp lime juice

3 tbsp plain yogurt, or coconut
    yogurt, or Blender Mayonnaise
    (see page 70)

sea salt and ground black pepper

steamed green beans or salad, to
    serve

**1** Preheat the oven to 200°C/400°F/Gas 6 and line a baking sheet with baking parchment, then lightly grease the paper. Put the egg in a bowl, add a pinch of sea salt and the sriracha sauce, and beat well.

**2** Put the red lentils into a blender or food processor and add the almond flour, garlic salt, paprika and onion powder. Whiz until fine, then tip onto a plate. Drop the chicken pieces into the egg and mix until fully covered. Lift the chicken pieces from the egg and into the flour mixture. Coat them evenly and then put them on the prepared baking sheet.

**3** Cook in the oven for 15 minutes, then flip the chicken over and cook for another 10 minutes or until golden and crispy.

**4** Meanwhile, put the avocado into a blender or food processor and add the garlic, lime juice and yogurt. Season with salt and pepper, then whiz to make the avocado mayonnaise. Serve the chicken with the mayo and green beans. (To freeze, open-freeze the uncooked, coated chicken bites, then pack and freeze for up to 3 months. Cook in the oven for 30–35 minutes from frozen.)

### Brain Benefits

Avocados are one of the best brain foods, rich in monounsaturated fats, which support the production of acetylcholine, the memory and learning brain chemical. They are an excellent source of vitamins that your brain needs, including C, E, K and B-complex vitamins. They also contain tyrosine, an amino acid that's a precursor to dopamine – the brain chemical that keeps you motivated and focused.

NUTRITIONAL INFORMATION PER SERVING 451 Kcals, **Protein** 35.6g, Carbohydrates 14.6g of which sugars 10.2g, **Fat** 26.2g of which saturates 8.7g

# Chicken Pad Thai

Almond butter, coconut milk, and the classic flavours of lime, garlic and ginger are balanced in this appetizing sauce quickly whizzed up in a blender. The recipe includes courgette/zucchini noodles, but you could also use kelp noodles, which are ready to eat after a quick rinse under warm water.

Serves 2
Preparation: 20 minutes
Cooking: 15 minutes

2 tbsp cashew nuts
2 sun-dried tomatoes in oil, drained
2 tsp lime juice
1 tsp fish sauce
½ garlic clove, peeled
1 tbsp tamari soy sauce
5mm/¼in piece of root ginger,
    peeled and grated
2 tbsp almond butter
1 tsp xylitol or erythritol
3–4 tbsp coconut milk, as needed
1 tbsp coconut oil
200g/7oz skinless chicken breast,
    cut into thin strips
2 courgettes/zucchini, spiralized, or
    150g/5½oz kelp noodles
1 carrot, cut into thin matchsticks
60g/2¼oz mangetout/snow peas,
    cut into strips lengthways
½ red pepper/bell pepper,
    deseeded and cut into thin strips
1 handful of fresh coriander/
    cilantro leaves, chopped
1 handful of fresh mint, chopped

**1** Put the nuts in a small saucepan and toast them over a medium-high heat for 1–2 minutes or until evenly toasted, shaking the pan frequently. Chop the nuts and leave to one side.

**2** Put the sun-dried tomatoes into a food processor and add the lime juice, fish sauce, garlic, tamari, ginger, almond butter, xylitol and 3 tablespoons of the milk. Whiz until the sauce is completely smooth, adding more milk if needed.

**3** Heat the oil in a large frying pan over a medium heat. Add the chicken and stir-fry for 2–3 minutes until lightly golden. Pour over the tomato mixture, bring to the boil, then reduce the heat and simmer gently for 7–8 minutes until the chicken is just cooked. Add the courgette/zucchini noodles to the pan with the carrot, mangetout/snow peas and red pepper/bell pepper. Cook over a medium heat for 1–2 minutes to soften slightly. Scatter over the herbs and serve.

### Brain Benefits

Almonds are loaded with nutrients such as vitamin B6, which promotes brain health, and vitamin E, which slows down the ageing of brain cells, thereby impacting memory. The kelp noodles (as an alternative to the spiralized courgettes/zucchini) are rich in iodine to support metabolism and cognitive function as well as being a great low-carb, gluten-free option to regular noodles.

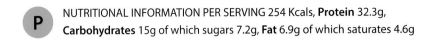

**P** NUTRITIONAL INFORMATION PER SERVING 254 Kcals, **Protein** 32.3g, **Carbohydrates** 15g of which sugars 7.2g, **Fat** 6.9g of which saturates 4.6g

# One-Pot Indian Chicken

Lightly fried chicken is bathed in fresh Indian flavours and makes a wonderful anti-inflammatory one-pot meal. Cauliflower rice (page 167) makes the perfect accompaniment.

Serves 2
Preparation: 15 minutes
Cooking: 23 minutes

250g/9oz boneless chicken thighs, cut into large chunks
2 tbsp cornflour/cornstarch
1–2 tbsp coconut oil
1 garlic clove, crushed
1 onion, cut in half and thinly sliced
1cm/½in piece of root ginger, peeled and grated
4 curry leaves
2 star anise
½ tsp curry powder or garam masala
½ tsp ground turmeric or 5mm/¼in piece of turmeric root, peeled and grated
1 tsp ground coriander
½ x 400g/14oz can full-fat coconut milk
2 large handfuls of baby spinach leaves
8 button mushrooms, cut in half
8 cherry tomatoes, cut in half
1 handful of coriander/cilantro leaves, chopped
sea salt and ground black pepper

**1** Dust the chicken pieces in cornflour/cornstarch and season with salt and pepper. Heat 1 tablespoon of the oil in a large saucepan over a low heat. When the oil is hot, add the chicken pieces and fry gently for 3 minutes or until they are lightly golden. Remove from the pan and leave to one side.

**2** Add a little more oil if needed, then add the garlic, onion and spices, and cook for 3 minutes or until the onion is translucent.

**3** Add the coconut milk, bring to the boil, then reduce the heat to a gentle simmer. Add the chicken, spinach, mushrooms and tomatoes. Simmer, uncovered, for 15 minutes or until the chicken is completely cooked through. Top with the coriander/cilantro and serve.

**Brain Benefits**

This dish contains healthy brain fats due to the addition of coconut oil and coconut milk. The combination of spices helps to lower inflammation in the body and protect the brain cells from free-radical damage. The curcumin in turmeric is able to cross the blood–brain barrier, and holds promise as a neuro-protective agent.

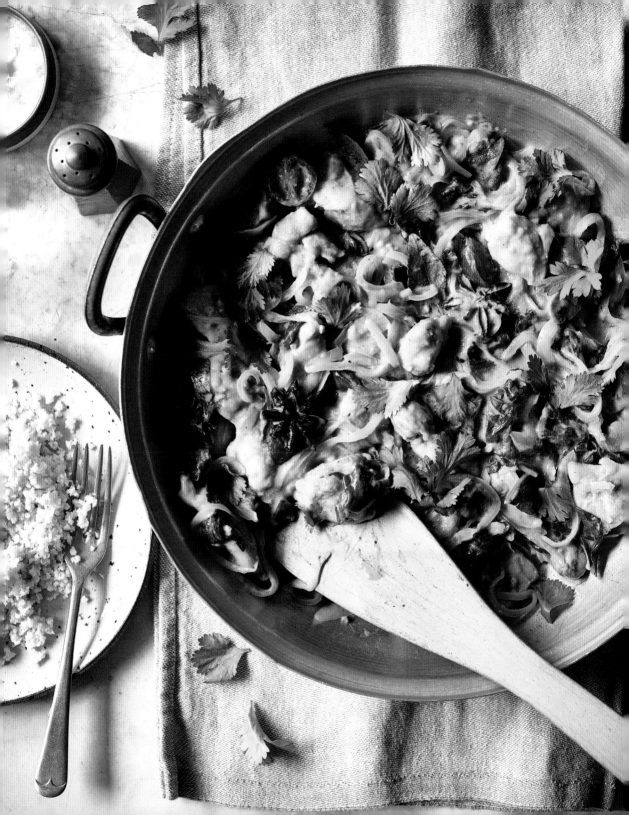

NUTRITIONAL INFORMATION PER SERVING 308 Kcals, **Protein** 29.2g,
**Carbohydrates** 17.2g of which sugars 7.2g, **Fat** 12.1g of which saturates 3.1g

# Soy-Braised Duck with Garlicky Leeks

A tangy soy and lemongrass marinade is combined with lightly cooked greens to make an energizing high-protein dish. The sourness of tamarind and lime complements the richness of the duck.

Serves 2
Preparation: 15 minutes, plus
    30 minutes marinating
Cooking: 20 minutes, plus
    5 minutes resting

2 boneless duck breasts, with skin
2 tsp fish sauce
2 tbsp tamari soy sauce
2 tsp xylitol or erythritol
2 garlic cloves, chopped
1 lemongrass stalk, outer leaves
    and top discarded
1 tbsp lime juice
1 tbsp tamarind paste
1 tsp tamari soy sauce
100ml/3½fl oz/scant ½ cup chicken
    or vegetable stock
2 tsp olive oil or coconut oil
3 leeks, cut in half and cut
    diagonally into 1cm/½in slices
sea salt and ground black pepper

**1** Using a sharp knife, score a crisscross pattern across the skin side of the duck breasts. Put in a shallow ovenproof dish and drizzle with the fish sauce, tamari and half the xylitol. Season with salt and pepper and put in the refrigerator for 30 minutes. Preheat the oven to 200°C/400°F/Gas 6.

**2** Put the garlic into a blender and add the lemon-grass, remaining xylitol, lime juice, tamarind, tamari and stock. Whiz until smooth.

**3** Heat the oil in a large saucepan over a medium heat, then add the leeks and toss to coat in the oil. Add the tamarind mixture and stir to cover the leeks. Reduce the heat, cover and cook gently for 20 minutes or until the leeks are tender.

**4** Meanwhile, drain the duck breasts and dry on paper towels. Heat an ovenproof frying pan over a medium-high heat until hot. Sear the duck on both sides, then reduce the heat to low and cook the fat side for 10 minutes or until most of the fat has rendered. Transfer the pan to the oven and cook for 10 minutes. Remove the duck from the oven and allow the meat to rest for 5 minutes, then slice very thinly. Serve the duck with the leeks.

### Brain Benefits
Leeks are part of the garlic and onion family that are all packed with antioxidants for staving off disease and eliminating free-radical damage. They are also a great addition for cleansing the body and providing prebiotics to support healthy gut bacteria. This dish also contains B vitamins, iron and zinc for healthy cognitive function.

NUTRITIONAL INFORMATION PER SERVING 485 Kcals, **Protein** 36.3g,
**Carbohydrates** 13.6g of which sugars 10.4g, **Fat** 29.5g of which saturates 5.1g

# Salmon Tataki

Tataki is a Japanese method of quickly searing fish or meat before chilling and slicing. It is normally dressed with a fragrant dressing. Try to find very fresh high-quality wild salmon for this dish. You could also use prawns/shrimp or squid. If you cannot find daikon, use ½ cucumber instead.

Serves 2
Preparation: 15 minutes, plus
   1–2 hours chilling
Cooking: 5 minutes

250g/9oz salmon fillet, boned and
   skinned
2 tbsp olive oil
2 tbsp sesame seeds
½ shallot, finely chopped
2 star anise
3 tbsp tamari soy sauce
2 tbsp rice vinegar
2 tbsp mirin
1 tsp xylitol or erythritol
5mm/¼in piece of root ginger,
   peeled and grated
1 tsp sesame oil
2 heads of pak choi/bok choy, cut
   in half lengthways, or 250g/9oz
   shredded Chinese cabbage
100g/3½oz daikon, peeled and cut
   into thin matchsticks, or grated
   or spiralized
sea salt and ground black pepper

**1** Cut the salmon fillet crossways in half, then drizzle the fish with 1 tbsp olive oil. Put the sesame seeds on a plate. Roll the salmon in the sesame seeds and season all over with salt and pepper.

**2** Heat a non-stick frying pan with a lid over a medium heat. Sear the fillets until lightly brown on all sides, this will take about 2 minutes. Leave to cool slightly, then put the salmon in cling film/plastic wrap and wrap tightly. Chill for 1, or ideally, 2 hours.

**3** Put the shallot in a bowl and add the star anise, tamari, vinegar, mirin, xylitol, ginger, sesame oil and remaining olive oil. Whisk together to make a dressing.

**4** Put the pak choi/bok choy in a frying pan over a medium heat with 1 tablespoon water and 2 tablespoons of the dressing. Cover the pan and steam-fry for 3 minutes or until the pak choi is just softened. Tip in the daikon and drizzle over a little more dressing to coat. Turn off the heat.

**5** Unwrap the fish and slice it very thinly. Divide between plates and drizzle with the remaining dressing. Serve with the pak choi and daikon.

### Brain Benefits

Daikon is known to support digestion, thanks to an enzyme called diastase, which helps to relieve indigestion and heartburn. It also contains isothiocyanates – giving daikon its peppery and pungent qualities – and these might help to improve blood circulation.

NUTRITIONAL INFORMATION PER SERVING 350 Kcals, **Protein** 35.6g,
**Carbohydrates** 23.5g of which sugars 11.4g, **Fat** 11.7g of which saturates 4.2g

# Sweet Potato Gratin Fish Pie

Fish pie is often a stodgy comfort dish, but this lighter version uses sweet potato and cauliflower to reduce carbohydrate and add antioxidants. For a dairy-free version, use coconut milk and omit the cheese.

**Serves 4**
**Preparation: 25 minutes**
**Cooking: 45 minutes**

100g/3½oz raw king prawns/jumbo
  shrimp
2 medium leeks, shredded
150g/5½oz smoked haddock fillet,
  boned and skinned
150g/5½oz cod fillet, boned and
  skinned
150g/5½oz salmon fillet, boned and
  skinned
500ml/17fl oz/2 cups semi-
  skimmed milk or canned full-fat
  coconut milk
1 tsp Dijon mustard
1 tbsp cornflour/cornstarch
zest of 1 lemon
1 tbsp chopped parsley leaves
1 tbsp chopped dill fronds
1 sweet potato, peeled
150g/5½oz cauliflower, cut into
  florets
1 tbsp olive oil
2 tbsp grated Parmesan cheese
sea salt and ground black pepper
green salad and lemon wedges, to
  serve

**1** Preheat the oven to 200°C/400°F/Gas 6. Make a shallow cut down the centre of the curved back of each prawn/shrimp. Pull out the black vein with a cocktail stick/toothpick or your fingers, then rinse the prawn thoroughly.

**2** Put the leeks in a large frying with a lid and add 1 tablespoon water. Cover and steam-fry over a medium heat for 5 minutes or until the leeks are soft. Add the fish, prawns, milk and mustard to the pan, return to the boil, then reduce the heat, cover and simmer for 5 minutes or until the fish is opaque and starting to flake and the prawns are pink. Drain and reserve the liquid, then remove the fish, prawns and leeks and put them into an ovenproof dish.

**3** Mix the cornflour/cornstarch with a little water to form a smooth paste. Stir into the hot milk liquid. Heat it gently, stirring well for 2 minutes or until the milk thickens. Season and add the lemon zest. Stir in the herbs, then pour over the fish and leeks.

**4** Meanwhile, put the whole peeled sweet potato into a large saucepan of boiling salted water and add the cauliflower florets. Blanch for 2 minutes. Remove from the pan, cool slightly, then grate the potato and cauliflower into a large, clean dish towel. Squeeze gently to remove the excess liquid. Tip the mixture into a bowl. Add the olive oil and Parmesan cheese, toss and season with salt and pepper. Scatter the mixture over the fish.

**5** Bake for 25–30 minutes until the top is golden brown and the filling bubbling hot. Serve with salad and lemon wedges. To freeze: make the fish pie in a freezerproof container and freeze for up to 3 months.

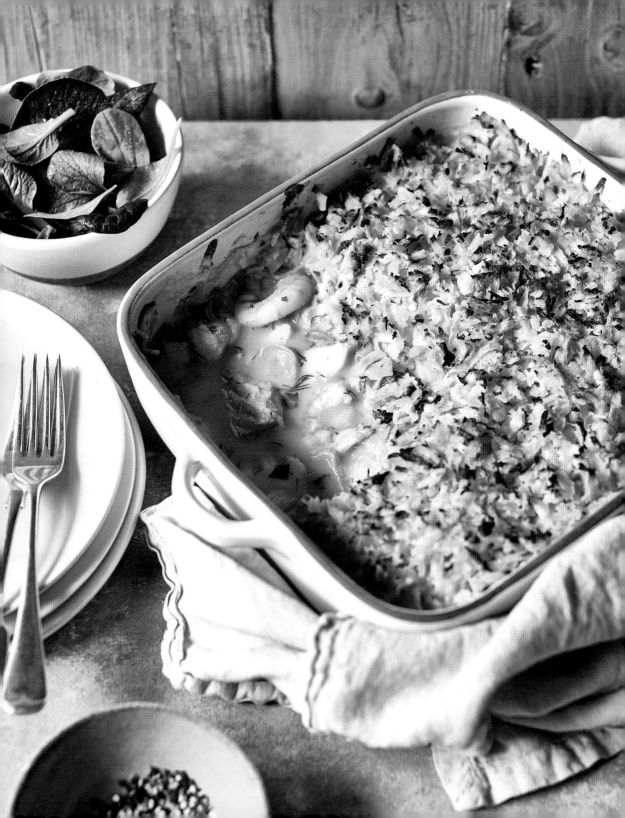

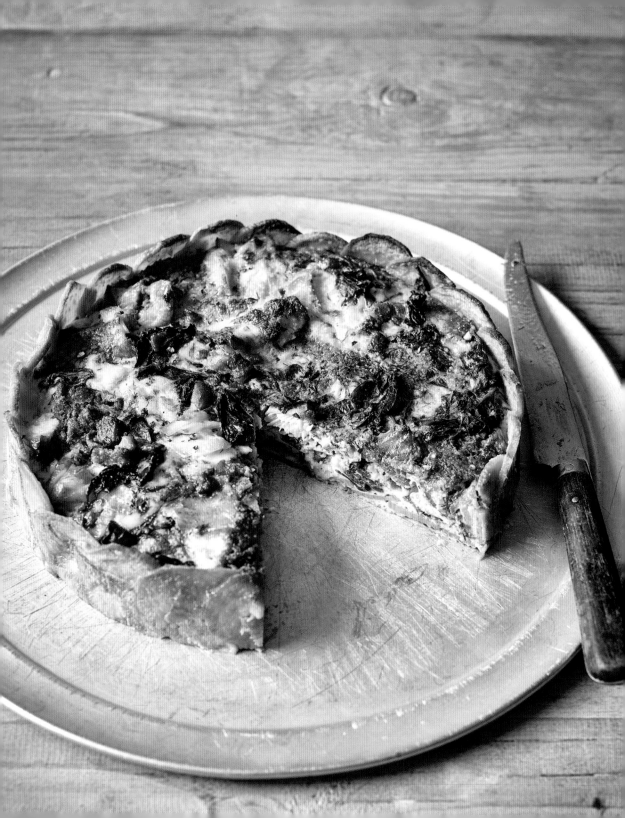

NUTRITIONAL INFORMATION PER SLICE 346 Kcals, **Protein** 20.4g,
**Carbohydrates** 14.2g of which sugars 4.3g, **Fat** 22.5g of which saturates 5.9g

# Hot-Smoked Salmon, Pancetta & Dill Pesto Tart

Using sweet potato slices rather than pastry gives a healthy, antioxidant-rich crust and adds even more flavour to the rich and creamy tart filling. It's a inspiring change from wheat-based tarts.

Makes 1 tart, 6 slices
Preparation: 20 minutes
Cooking: 35 minutes, plus
    10 minutes resting

1 tbsp coconut oil, plus extra for
    greasing
2 small sweet potatoes, sliced very
    thinly
60g/2¼oz pancetta, cubed
100g/3½oz baby spinach leaves,
    chopped
2 hot-smoked salmon fillets,
    200g/7oz total weight, skinned
7 eggs
sea salt and ground black pepper

FOR THE PESTO
½ garlic clove, chopped
2 tbsp toasted pine nuts
1 handful of flat-leaf parsley leaves,
    roughly chopped
1 handful of dill fronds, roughly
    chopped, plus extra to garnish
15g/½oz Parmesan, finely grated,
    or 2 tbsp nutritional yeast flakes
4 tbsp extra virgin olive oil
1 tbsp lemon juice

**1** Preheat the oven to 200°C/400°F/gas 6 and grease a 20cm/8in springform cake pan. Heat the oil in a saucepan over a medium-high heat and lightly fry the sweet potato slices in batches for 2–3 minutes until soft. Remove from the pan and leave to cool.

**2** Add the pancetta to the pan followed by the spinach and cook for 2 minutes or until the pancetta is golden and the spinach has wilted. Flake the salmon into chunks. Leave to one side.

**3** To make the pesto, whiz the garlic and pine nuts in a mini food processor. Add the parsley and dill, then pulse until finely chopped. Add the remaining ingredients to make a thick pesto – you might need to add a dash of water to combine.

**4** Line the base and sides of the prepared cake pan with the sweet potato, overlapping the slices so that there are no gaps.

**5** Beat the eggs with the pesto, season, and add the pancetta, spinach and salmon. Pour into the pan and bake for 30 minutes or until firm and golden. Leave to rest for 10 minutes before serving.

### Brain Benefits

Sweet potato is a rich source of vitamins A and C: antioxidants that protect neurons as well as providing soluble fibre to support a healthy gut. Being low on the glycaemic list they won't disrupt your blood sugar levels either.

# Perfect Pestos

I absolutely love making my own pesto. It's simple to make, perfect for preparing in a large batch, freezes well, and is a great way of getting more greens in the diet. I like to vary the greens, herbs and nuts according to what's in the house. I like cashew nuts because they are so creamy, but macadamia nuts add more oleic acid – the same fat found in olive oil and good for the myelin sheath (the fatty layer that insulates and protects nerve cells in the brain). Try other nuts too, such as walnuts, pistachio nuts and almonds. If you have time, soak the nuts in water for 1–2 hours, then drain before using. This makes them easy to digest and creates a creamier texture.  Make of any the recipes that include Parmesan dairy-free, and so Paleo or vegan, by substiting the cheese for nutritional yeast flakes.

*These pestos are simple to make and a great way of getting more greens into your diet.*

## Broccoli Pesto

 **V**   NUTRITIONAL INFORMATION PER 1 TBSP 32 Kcals, **Protein** 1.2g, **Carbohydrates** 0.6g of which sugars 0.3g, **Fat** 2.7g of which saturates 0.6g

MAKES about 480g/1lb 1oz/2 cups  PREPARATION: 10 minutes  COOKING: 3 minutes

✛1 small head of broccoli (about 300g/10½oz), cut into florets  ✛1 large handful of basil leaves  ✛2 garlic cloves, chopped  ✛juice of ½ lemon  ✛30g/1oz/¼ cup macadamia nuts  ✛50g/1¾oz/scant 1 cup cashew nuts  ✛2 tbsp grated Parmesan cheese or nutritional yeast flakes  ✛3–4 tbsp olive oil to blend or a combination of MCT oil and olive oil  ✛sea salt and ground black pepper

**1** Steam the broccoli florets over a saucepan of boiling water for 2–3 minutes until just soft. Put into a blender or food processor, and add the basil, garlic, lemon juice, nuts and Parmesan. Blend while gradually adding the oil until you have a smooth and creamy pesto. Season with salt and pepper to taste.
**2** Transfer to a sealable glass jar and store in the refrigerator for 1 week or freeze for up to 3 months.

**Brain Benefits**
Broccoli is a source of vitamin K, which helps to strengthen cognitive abilities, and choline, which has been found to improve memory. It also includes folic acid, which can help to ward off Alzheimer's disease. Studies suggest a lack of folic acid could also lead to depression, so eating plenty of broccoli might also keep you happy.

# Super Kale Pesto

 **V** NUTRITIONAL INFORMATION PER 1 TBSP 44 Kcals, **Protein** 1.5g, **Carbohydrates** 0.2g of which sugars 0.2g, **Fat** 4g of which saturates 0.8g

MAKES 360g/12¾oz/1½ cups PREPARATION: 10 minutes COOKING: 2 minutes

✣ 75g/2½oz/½ cup walnuts ✣ 2 garlic cloves, peeled ✣ 180g/6¼oz kale, chopped ✣ juice of ½ lemon ✣ 50g/1¾oz/ scant 1 cup grated Parmesan cheese or 3 tbsp nutritional yeast flakes ✣ 3–4 tbsp olive oil or a combination of MCT and olive oil ✣ sea salt and ground black pepper

**1** Put the walnuts in a small saucepan and toast them over a medium-high heat for 1–2 minutes or until evenly toasted, shaking the pan frequently.
**2** Put the walnuts, garlic, kale, lemon juice and Parmesan into a food processor. Blend while gradually adding the oil until you have a smooth and creamy pesto. Store in an airtight container in the refrigerator for up to 1 week or freeze for up to 3 months.

### Brain Benefits
Walnuts are one of the best nuts for brain health, as they are a good source of plant-based omega-3 fats and antioxidants, which can help to prevent or ameliorate age-related cognitive decline. The antioxidants can even reduce the risk of neurodegenerative diseases, including Alzheimer's.

# Roasted Macadamia Tomato Pesto

 **P**  **V**  **VE** NUTRITIONAL INFORMATION PER 1 TBSP 103 Kcals, **Protein** 0.5g, **Carbohydrates** 0.4g of which sugars 0.2g, **Fat** 11.1g of which saturates 1.6g

MAKES 280g/10oz/scant 1¼ cups PREPARATION: 10 minutes COOKING: 2 minutes

✣ 70g/2½oz/½ cup macadamia nuts ✣ 60g/2¼oz sun-dried tomatoes in oil, drained and chopped ✣ 1 garlic clove ✣ 2 tbsp lemon juice ✣ 1 large handful of basil leaves ✣ 125ml/4fl oz/½ cup olive oil or macadamia oil, or use the oil from the sun-dried tomato jar

**1** Put the macadamia nuts in a small saucepan and lightly toast over a medium-high heat for 1–2 minutes until just starting to turn colour.
**2** Put all the ingredients into a blender or food processor and whiz to form a thick paste. Store in the refrigerator for up to 2 weeks or freeze for up to 3 months.

### Brain Benefits
I like to use macademia nuts for this creamy pesto, as they are rich in oleic acid, which is beneficial for health because of its anti-inflammatory properties and for supporting the brain-cell membranes.

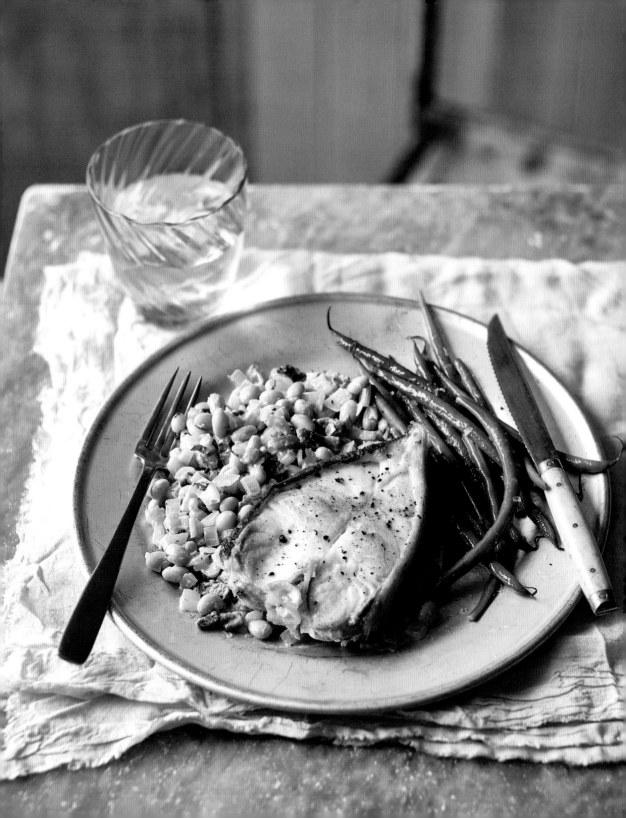

NUTRITIONAL INFORMATION PER SERVING 413 Kcals, **Protein** 36.9g,
**Carbohydrates** 22.9g of which sugars 4.2g, **Fat** 16.3g of which saturates 8g

# Pan-Fried Halibut with Haricot Beans

This simple, French-inspired dish is packed with flavours and is very quick to make using canned haricot beans for speed. The yogurt adds a lovely creamy texture to the sauce.

Serves 2
Preparation: 15 minutes
Cooking: 12 minutes, plus 5
   minutes resting

2 halibut fillets, 120g/4¼oz each,
   skinned
1 tbsp olive oil
2 celery stalks, finely chopped
1 garlic clove, crushed
½ onion, chopped
2 slices of smoked back/lean bacon,
   cut into small pieces
400g/14oz can haricot/navy beans
   or cannellini beans, drained and
   rinsed
1 tarragon sprig, leaves chopped
zest of ½ lemon
1 tbsp coconut oil
200g/7oz green beans
2 tbsp coconut yogurt or Greek
   yogurt
sea salt

**1** Remove the halibut fillets from the refrigerator and allow to come to room temperature before cooking. Preheat the oven to 180°C/350°F/Gas 4. Heat the oil in a saucepan and fry the celery, garlic, onion and bacon for 2–3 minutes until the bacon is golden brown and lightly crisp, stirring frequently. Remove from the heat and tip in the haricot/navy beans, tarragon and lemon zest.

**2** Season the halibut well with salt, then heat the coconut oil in an ovenproof frying pan until hot. Add the fish and cook for 2 minutes or until lightly golden.

**3** Transfer the pan to the oven and cook for 5 minutes. After this time, remove from the oven, turn the fillets over and allow them to rest, off the heat, for 5 minutes – the residual heat from the pan should cook the fillets through.

**4** Meanwhile, bring a saucepan of water to the boil and blanch the green beans for 2–3 minutes until al dente, then drain well.

**5** Heat through the bean and bacon mixture. Add the yogurt to the pan and toss briefly to heat through. Serve the halibut with the bean mixture and the green beans alongside.

### Brain Benefits
Halibut is an excellent source of omega-3 fats plus protein and vitamin B12 – two nutrients to support a healthy brain.

NUTRITIONAL INFORMATION PER SERVING 499 Kcals, **Protein** 36.7g,
**Carbohydrates** 48.8g of which sugars 5.3g, **Fat** 15.9g of which saturates 9.1g

# Spiced Fish Fingers & Tartare Peas

The probiotic-rich coleslaw makes the perfect accompaniment for crispy fried fish coated with a combination of oats and polenta/cornmeal. It is served alongside my creamy and tangy tartare peas – an unusual and incredibly tasty way to jazz up frozen peas. Serve with a green salad as well, if you like.

Serves 2

Preparation: 20 minutes, plus
    making the sauerkraut and mayo
Cooking: 15 minutes

60g/2¼oz/scant ⅔ cup gluten-free
    oats
½ tsp ground turmeric
½ tsp ground cumin
¼ tsp smoked paprika
80g/2¾oz polenta/cornmeal
1 egg
250g/9oz cod or haddock fillet,
    skinned and cut into
    chunky strips
2 tbsp coconut oil
100g/3½oz/⅔ cup Coleslaw
    Sauerkraut (page 67)
sea salt and ground black pepper

**FOR THE TARTARE PEAS**
100g/3½oz/¾ cup frozen peas
3 tbsp yogurt or Blender
    Mayonnaise (see page 70)
2 tsp gherkins, finely chopped
2 tsp capers, drained, rinsed and
    finely chopped
2 tsp finely chopped shallots
2 tsp finely chopped parsley leaves

**1** Put the oats and spices into a food processor and whiz until it is like a fine flour. Tip onto a plate and stir in the polenta/cornmeal. Put the egg in a shallow bowl and beat in a little salt.

**2** Dip a strip of fish into the egg, then coat in the oat mixture. Make sure that it is coated all over. Repeat with all the fish strips.

**3** Heat the oil in a frying pan over a medium-high heat and put in a few of the fish fingers. Cook for 2–3 minutes until the edges turn golden. Carefully turn over and cook for another 1–2 minutes until golden brown all over. Remove from the pan and keep warm. Repeat with the remaining fish fingers.

**4** Meanwhile, to make the tartare peas, bring a saucepan of water to the boil and blanch the peas for 2–3 minutes until just cooked. Drain in a colander. Put the remaining tartare ingredients in a bowl. Mix together well, then add the peas and stir well. Serve the fish with the coleslaw and tartare peas.

**Brain Benefits**
Green peas are a great source of fibre to support cleansing and detoxification. They're also rich in B vitamins, including the folates, which are required for DNA synthesis and keeping homocysteine levels healthy (see page 9). They also provide the carotenoids and the antioxidants, catechin and epicatechin, plus many polyphenols known for their anti-inflammatory properties.

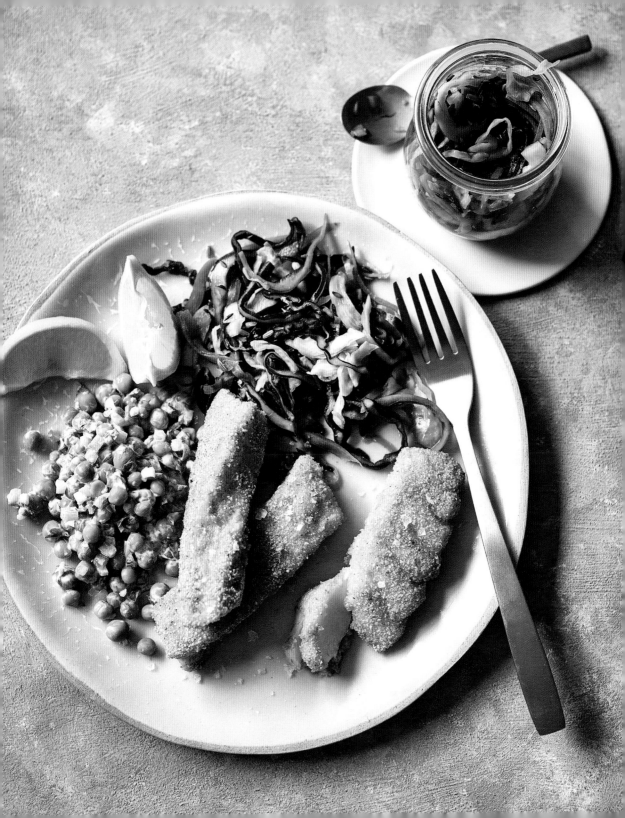

**P** NUTRITIONAL INFORMATION PER SERVING 473 Kcals, **Protein** 40.7g, **Carbohydrates** 6.2g of which sugars 5g, **Fat** 31.2g of which saturates 5g

# Sardines with 5-Minute Romesco Sauce

Quick and easy, this version of the Spanish Romesco sauce is pure magic. You can use it as a marinade, a condiment or a dip – or just eat it with a spoon! It's a great addition to any grilled/broiled fish or seafood.

Serves 2
Preparation: 15 minutes
Cooking: 6 minutes

60g/2¼oz/½ cup almonds
120g/4¼oz/1 large roasted red
 pepper/bell pepper from a jar,
 drained
1 handful of basil leaves
1 garlic clove, peeled
2 tomatoes, cut in half and seeds
 removed
1 tbsp red wine vinegar
1 tbsp olive oil
a pinch of dried chilli/hot pepper
 flakes (optional)
1 tsp finely grated lemon zest
1 tbsp finely chopped parsley
 leaves
1 garlic clove, very finely chopped
1½ tsp finely chopped pitted green
 olives
1½ tsp capers, drained, rinsed and
 chopped
extra virgin olive oil, for greasing
 and drizzling
4 sardines, cleaned and trimmed
sea salt and ground black pepper
lemon wedges, to serve

**1** Put the almonds into a blender or food processor and add the red pepper/bell pepper, basil, garlic, tomatoes, vinegar, olive oil and dried chilli/hot pepper flakes, if using. Season with salt and pepper and whiz to form a smooth, thick Romesco sauce.

**2** Put the lemon zest in a bowl and add the parsley, chopped garlic, olives and capers, season and mix together.

**3** Preheat the grill/broiler to high and lightly grease a baking sheet. Lay the sardines on the prepared sheet and sprinkle with extra virgin olive oil, salt and pepper. Grill/broil for 2–3 minutes on each side or until cooked through. Serve the sardines scattered with the parsley mixture, accompanied with the Romesco sauce and lemon wedges.

## Brain Benefits

Red peppers/bell peppers are one of the best sources of the red-coloured carotenoid pigment, lycopene, and of lutein and zeaxanthin, which are potent antioxidants for the brain. They also provide vitamin B6, which plays an important role in brain function and the production of neurotransmitters.

P NUTRITIONAL INFORMATION PER SERVING 350 Kcals, **Protein** 26.1g, **Carbohydrates** 9g of which sugars 5.4g, **Fat** 22.2g of which saturates 5.8g

# Grilled Sea Bass with Caponata

A delicious prepare-ahead Mediterranean dish, caponata is a luscious Italian vegetable melange that goes very well with flavourful sea bass. You can serve the caponata warm or at room temperature, and it is also delicious topped with grilled/broiled chicken as an alternative.

**Serves 4**
**Preparation: 20 minutes**
**Cooking: 30 minutes**

2 aubergines/eggplants, cut into cubes
3 tbsp olive oil
1 small red onion, diced
2 garlic cloves, crushed
1 anchovy in oil, drained
2 x 400g/14oz cans plum tomatoes, chopped
1 red pepper/bell pepper, deseeded and cut into 1cm/½in pieces
4 celery stalks, cut into 1cm/½in pieces
4 tbsp white wine vinegar
1 tbsp tomato purée/paste
2 tbsp capers, drained and rinsed
10 pitted green olives
1 tbsp xylitol or erythritol
4 sea bass fillets (skin on)
1 tbsp coconut oil
juice of ½ lemon
sea salt and ground black pepper

**1** Preheat the oven to 200°C/400°F/Gas 6. Put the aubergine/eggplant pieces in a roasting pan, drizzle over 2 tablespoons of the olive oil and season with salt and pepper. Cook in the oven for 20 minutes or until golden and tender.

**2** Meanwhile, heat the remaining olive oil in a large saucepan over a medium heat and cook the onion, garlic, anchovy and tomatoes for 10 minutes, breaking up the tomatoes as they cook. Add the red pepper/bell pepper, celery, vinegar, tomato purée/paste, capers, olives and xylitol. Add the aubergine, then cover and cook for 10 minutes or until the pepper and celery are soft and the caponata mixture is thick.

**3** Meanwhile, season the sea bass fillets with salt and pepper. Heat the coconut oil in an ovenproof frying pan. Put the fillets into the pan, skin-side down, and cook for 3 minutes or until the skin is crispy, then put the frying pan in the oven for 4 minutes. Drizzle over the lemon juice. Serve the sea bass with the caponata.

### Brain Benefits

Sea bass is high in protein, which is needed for the production of brain neurotransmitters, and healthy fats for optimum brain function. It is also rich in the antioxidant selenium, plus vitamins B12 and B6 to support neurotransmitter production. The caponata is packed with protective brain antioxidants.

**P** NUTRITIONAL INFORMATION PER SERVING 535 Kcals, **Protein** 23.8g, **Carbohydrates** 26.5g of which sugars 20.4g, **Fat** 36.3g of which saturates 6.8g

# Pomegranate-Glazed Mackerel with Roasted Fennel

The delicious Iranian condiment, pomegranate molasses, is a made from boiled, crushed pomegranate seeds and has a sweet tangy flavour. It is perfect for salad dressings or made into marinades for meat and fish.

Serves 2
Preparation: 15 minutes
Cooking: 30 minutes

1 fennel bulb, cut into thick wedges
8 cherry tomatoes
1 tsp fennel seeds
1 tbsp olive oil, plus extra for greasing
2 tbsp pomegranate molasses
1 garlic clove, crushed
2 mackerel fillets, boned with skin
salad leaves/greens and pomegranate seeds, to serve

FOR THE DRESSING
2 tbsp pomegranate molasses
1 tbsp lemon juice
¼ tsp ground cumin
½ garlic clove, crushed
2 tbsp extra virgin olive oil or flaxseed/omega-3-rich oil
sea salt and ground black pepper

1 Preheat the oven to 160°C/315°F/Gas 2½. Put the fennel in a roasting pan, then scatter over the tomatoes and fennel seeds. Season with salt and pepper and drizzle with the olive oil and add a splash of water. Cook in the oven for 30 minutes or until the fennel is tender and caramelized.

2 Meanwhile, put the pomegranate molasses in a bowl and add the garlic, then season and mix well. Rub this all over the mackerel fillets.

3 Put all the dressing ingredients in a screwtop jar and add 1 tablespoon water, then shake well to combine. Leave to one side.

4 Preheat the grill/broiler to high and line a baking sheet with foil. Grease the foil lightly. Put the mackerel fillets on the prepared baking sheet and grill/broil for 4–5 minutes, or until the skin turns golden and brown and the flesh firms up. Season. Serve the fish with salad, and drizzle over the dressing and scatter with pomegranate seeds. Serve with the braised fennel.

### Brain Benefits

Pomegranates contain an impressive amount of antioxidants and provide a good source of B vitamins, copper, manganese, fibre and phosphorus, that together might boost your brain health and protect the brain from free-radical damage.

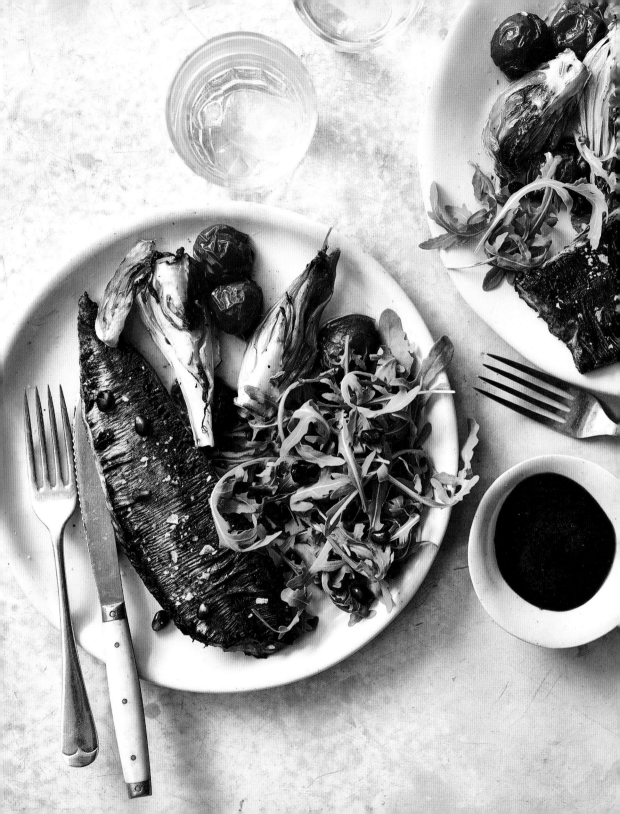

NUTRITIONAL INFORMATION PER SERVING 215 Kcals, **Protein** 25.4g, **Carbohydrates** 17g of which sugars 13.8g, **Fat** 3.4g of which saturates 0.9g

# Light Prawn Laksa

Laksa is a Peranakan dish originating in Malaysia, and popular in Singapore and Thailand. This version has a rich broth with anti-inflammatory spices and coconut milk. Although there are a lot of ingredients, this is actually very quick and easy to make.

Serves 2

Preparation: 20 minutes

Cooking: 10 minutes, plus
    5 minutes standing

2 garlic cloves, chopped

2cm/¾in piece of root ginger,
    peeled and chopped

½ red chilli, deseeded

½ tsp ground turmeric or 5mm/¼in
    turmeric root, peeled and grated

2 spring onions/scallions

1 lemongrass stalk, trimmed

1 tsp peanut or almond butter

1 tbsp tamari soy sauce

2 tsp fish sauce

1 tsp xylitol or erythritol

1 tsp tomato purée/paste

200g/7oz raw king prawns/jumbo
    shrimp, peeled

300ml/10½fl oz/scant 1⅓ cups
    chicken stock

8 asparagus spears, cut in half

4 shiitake mushrooms, sliced

400ml/14fl oz/1¾ cups coconut milk

250g/9oz celeriac, sweet potato or
    courgette/zucchini, spiralized

**1** Put the garlic into a food processor and add the ginger, chilli, turmeric, spring onions/scallions, lemongrass, peanut butter, tamari, fish sauce, xylitol and tomato purée/paste. Whiz to form a paste – you may need to scrape down the side of the food processor to incorporate all the ingredients.

**2** Make a shallow cut down the centre of the curved back of each prawn/shrimp. Pull out the black vein with a cocktail stick/toothpick or your fingers, then rinse the prawn thoroughly. Leave to one side.

**3** Heat the stock in a saucepan over a medium-high heat and add the spice paste. Bring to the boil, then reduce the heat and simmer for 5 minutes. Add the asparagus to the pan, followed by the mushrooms and prawns, then pour in the milk. Bring to the boil, then reduce the heat and simmer for 3 minutes or until the prawns are pink and cooked.

**4** Turn off the heat, then add the celeriac to the pan. Allow the mixture to stand for 5 minutes before serving.

---

### Brain Benefits

Prawns/shrimp are protein-rich and contain healthy doses of vitamin B12 and omega-3 fatty acids, both of which are known to protect the ageing brain from cognitive decline.

---

**P** NUTRITIONAL INFORMATION PER SERVING 205 Kcals, **Protein** 26.8g, **Carbohydrates** 3.1g of which sugars 2.8g, **Fat** 9g of which saturates 1.6g

# Vegetable Spaghetti with Mussels

Here's how to create a Mediterranean feast in minutes! Based on the classic Italian dish, this version uses courgette/zucchini pasta rather than spaghetti tossed with fresh mussels to make the ultimate healthy fast food. This also makes use of some storecupboard ingredients.

Serves 2
Preparation: 25 minutes
Cooking: 10 minutes

400g/14oz mussels in their shells
100ml/3½fl oz/scant ½ cup
    vegetable stock or white wine
1 tbsp olive oil
4 garlic cloves, crushed
1–2 pinches of dried chilli/hot
    pepper flakes, to taste
10 cherry tomatoes, quartered
2 courgettes/zucchini, spiralized
1 handful of fresh parsley leaves,
    roughly chopped
juice of ½ lemon
sea salt

**1** Scrub the mussels' shells under cold water. Discard any mussels that remain open after being sharply tapped. Scrape off the beards. Rinse well. Put the mussels in a large saucepan and add the vegetable stock. Cover and put over a medium heat, and steam for 3–4 minutes until the shells have opened. Remove from the pan and discard any that remain closed. Strain and reserve the cooking juices.

**2** Heat the oil in a large frying pan, then fry the garlic, dried chilli/hot pepper flakes and tomatoes for 1 minute or until the garlic turns lightly golden. Add the reserved mussel liquid, then simmer, uncovered, for 3 minutes or until you have a thin sauce and the tomatoes are soft.

**3** Add the courgette/zucchini to the pan, and return the mussels. Stir well so that everything is combined, then scatter over the parsley and add the lemon juice. Season with salt and serve in bowls.

### Brain Benefits

Mussels are a perfect brain food because they are packed with DHA and vitamin B12: two key nutrients that are vital to protecting your brain health and preserving your memory as you age. They also contain some trace minerals on which a healthy, happy brain depends.

NUTRITIONAL INFORMATION PER SERVING 546 Kcals, **Protein** 33g, **Carbohydrates** 18.2g of which sugars 15.2g, **Fat** 35.6g of which saturates 10.8g

# Quick & Spicy Mackerel Nasi Goreng

Save on the washing up with this speedy one-pot supper. Using smoked mackerel provides omega-3 fats. Sambal oelek is made with lots of red chillies, garlic, shallots and lime – vary according to how spicy you like it. Cultured vegetables such as sauerkraut and kimchi (pages 67 and 68) are good with this dish.

Serves 2
Preparation: 15 minutes
Cooking: 20 minutes

150g/5½oz cauliflower, roughly
    chopped
2 slices of smoked back/lean bacon,
    cut into 2cm/¾in pieces
1 tbsp coconut oil
2 spring onions/scallions, thinly
    sliced
1 tbsp sambal oelek or other chilli
    paste, or to taste
1 garlic clove, crushed
2 small carrots, grated
½ Chinese cabbage, shredded,
    or a 250g/9oz bag of stir-fry
    vegetables
2 smoked mackerel fillets, skinned
    and broken into large pieces
1 large handful of bean sprouts
1 tbsp yacon syrup or rice malt
    syrup
2 tbsp tamari soy sauce
2 tsp fish sauce
2 eggs
ground black pepper
lime wedges, to serve

**1** Put the cauliflower in a food processor, or electric chopper, and whiz until it resembles rice-like grains. Leave to one side.

**2** Heat a wok or large frying pan over a medium-high heat. Add the bacon to the pan and stir-fry for 2 minutes or until the bacon is golden and crispy. Transfer the bacon to a plate.

**3** Add the oil to the pan, then add the spring onions/scallions, sambal oelek, garlic, carrots and cabbage. Stir-fry for 2 minutes to soften the vegetables. Return the bacon to the pan and add the mackerel, bean sprouts, yacon syrup, tamari and fish sauce. Cook for 3–4 minutes until warmed through. Season with pepper.

**4** Tip in the cauliflower rice and warm through. Make two wells in the centre of the wok and crack in the eggs. Cover the pan and cook for 10 minutes or until the egg whites are nearly set. Serve with lime wedges.

**Brain Benefits**

Mackerel is among the top fish on the list for omega-3 content. It is also an important source of protein and B vitamins, particularly vitamin B12, which is particularly beneficial for keeping levels of homocysteine (see page 9) healthy and supporting the production of brain chemicals to boost mood and alertness.

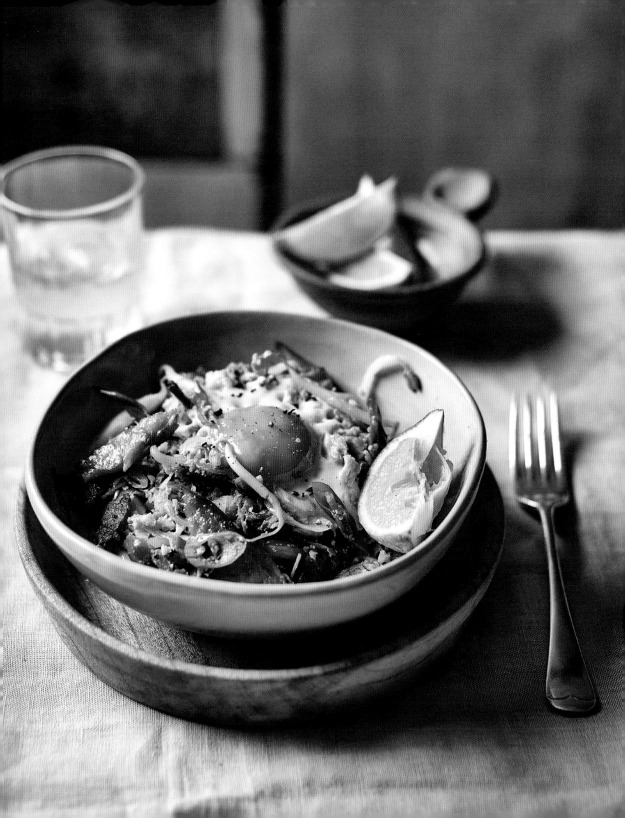

NUTRITIONAL INFORMATION PER SERVING 322 Kcals, **Protein** 33.4g,
**Carbohydrates** 31.1g of which sugars 22.3g, **Fat** 4.7g of which saturates 1g

# Indonesian Fish Curry with Cauliflower Rice

**Creamy and mild in flavour, my hearty halibut curry is packed with brain-friendly ingredients. Cauliflower rice goes wonderfully with it and is so much healthier than regular rice.**

Serves 2
Preparation: 15 minutes, plus
 1 hour or overnight marinating
Cooking: 7 minutes

200g/7oz halibut fillet, skinned and
 cut into large pieces
1 lemongrass stalk, chopped
1 handful of coriander/cilantro leaves
1 onion, chopped
2 garlic cloves, crushed
2cm/¾in piece of root ginger,
 peeled and chopped
2 tsp xylitol or erythritol or 1 tsp
 granulated stevia
1 tbsp tamari soy sauce
1 tsp fish sauce, or to taste
½ tsp ground turmeric or 5mm/¼in
 piece of root turmeric, peeled
 and grated
1 tsp garam masala
400g/14oz can full-fat coconut milk
2 tsp coconut oil
1 head of pak choi/bok choy, cut
 into strips
100g/3½oz mangetout/snow peas
4 shiitake mushrooms, sliced
2 spring onions/scallions, chopped
1 x quantity Cauliflower Rice (see
 page 167), to serve

**1** Put the fish in a shallow dish. Put the lemongrass into a blender or food processor and add the coriander/cilantro, onion, garlic, ginger, xylitol, tamari, fish sauce, turmeric, garam masala and milk. Whiz until smooth, then pour over the fish. Leave in the refrigerator to marinate for 1 hour.

**2** Heat the oil in a wok or frying pan. Add the pak choi/bok choy, mangetout/snow peas and mushrooms, and cook for 1 minute. Add the marinade and the fish pieces, and simmer for 5–6 minutes until the fish is cooked through. Scatter over the spring onions/scallions and serve with cauliflower rice.

### Brain Benefits

The anti-inflammatory ingredients in this dish include ginger, garlic and turmeric, together with immune-supporting shiitake mushrooms and coconut. Coconut milk is a good source of medium-chain triglycerides, which can be used by the brain for fuel as well as containing a wealth of minerals for energy production, including manganese, copper, magnesium, iron and potassium.

# Vegetable Rices

An easy way to reduce your overall carb intake and increase the vegetables in your diet is to use them to make rice. It's so quick and easy to prepare – all you need is a standard food processor with an S-blade or an electric food chopper. They are ideal for salads or to replace any grains in dishes. Although you can eat vegetable rices raw, they are equally delicious lightly cooked. In some of the recipes in this book, you will see the raw rice is simply added as part of the recipe, but it makes a great side to any dish.

## Cauliflower or Broccoli Rice

 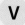  NUTRITIONAL INFORMATION PER SERVING (cauliflower) 38 Kcals, **Protein** 2.8g, **Carbohydrates** 4.7g of which sugars 3.1g, **Fat** 0.5g of which saturates 0.1g

SERVES 4 PREPARATION: 5 minutes

✜ 1 head of cauliflower or broccoli, about about 450g/1lb, roughly chopped (you can include the stalk) ✜ 1 tbsp olive oil, ghee or coconut oil (optional) ✜ herbs or spices, to taste (optional) ✜ sea salt and ground black pepper

**1** Put the cauliflower in a food processor and pulse until it forms rice-like grains. Store in the refrigerator for up to 4 days or freeze for up to 3 months.
**2** If cooking, heat the oil in a large frying pan. Stir in the vegetable rice and sprinkle with seasoning, herbs or spices to taste. Stir briefly. Cover and cook over a low heat for 3–4 minutes to allow the vegetable to steam-fry until it is soft. Serve immediately or use cold in salads. Store the cooked rice in the refrigerator for up to 4 days.

## VARIATION: PARSNIP OR CELERIAC RICE

➤ Any root vegetable can be used to make a rice, but parsnip or celeriac is particularly good. Yam and sweet potato also make tasty rices. This rice can be used in the nori rolls on page 131 to replace the cauliflower rice option. Put 4 large peeled parsnips or ½ peeled celeriac, roughly chopped, into a food processor, or electric chopper, with a pinch of sea salt and pulse until it resembles rice-like grains. Store in the refrigerator for up to 4 days or freeze for up to 3 months. Cook as above.

# Quinoa Bibimbap

**Serve this delicious vegetarian dish either in Chinese lettuce leaves or spooned into bowls. This version uses quinoa – a nourishing seed that contains protein – plus nutrient-rich eggs, nori and avocado.**

Serves 2
Preparation: 15 minutes
Cooking: 20 minutes, plus
    5 minutes standing

90g/3¼oz/½ cup quinoa
240ml/9fl oz/1 cup vegetable stock
1 tbsp coconut oil, plus extra if
    needed
½ onion, chopped
2 garlic cloves, crushed
4 shiitake mushrooms, thinly sliced
100g/3½oz baby spinach leaves
30g/1oz/heaping ¼ cup bean
    sprouts
3 tbsp tamari soy sauce
2 tsp granulated stevia, or xylitol
    or erythritol
2 tbsp rice wine vinegar
5mm/¼in piece of root ginger,
    peeled and grated
2 hard-boiled eggs, shelled, or
    poached eggs
½ ripe avocado, pitted, skinned and
    sliced or diced
1 sheet nori, crumbled
1 tbsp toasted sesame seeds
Chinese leaves, separated
Kimchi (page 68), to serve

**1** Rinse the quinoa well, then put it in a saucepan over a high heat and pour over the vegetable stock. Bring to the boil, then reduce the heat and simmer for 15 minutes or until tender. Turn off the heat and leave to steam for a further 5 minutes. Tip onto a plate lined with paper towels and pat dry.

**2** Heat the oil in a frying pan. Tip in the quinoa and fry for 1–2 minutes until the grains are slightly crisp and smell nutty. Add a little more oil, if needed, and add the onion, garlic, mushrooms, spinach, bean sprouts, tamari, stevia, vinegar and ginger. Stir-fry for 2–3 minutes until the spinach has wilted.

**3** Divide the quinoa mixture between two bowls. Top with the eggs, avocado, nori and sesame seeds. Alternatively, if spooning into Chinese leaves, chop the hard-boiled eggs, and stir into the mixture followed by the avocado and nori. Spoon the mixture into the Chinese leaves and scatter with sesame seeds. Serve with kimchi.

### Brain Benefits

Quinoa is a high-protein pseudo-grain rich in flavonoids, including quercetin and kaempferol, known for their potent antioxidant properties. It also provides a good source of the minerals iron and magnesium and, with a low glycaemic index (GI), it won't disrupt your blood sugar levels. The eggs contain beneficial brain fats, choline and protein, and the avocado is a rich source of monounsaturated fats and vitamin E, both of which are excellent for brain health.

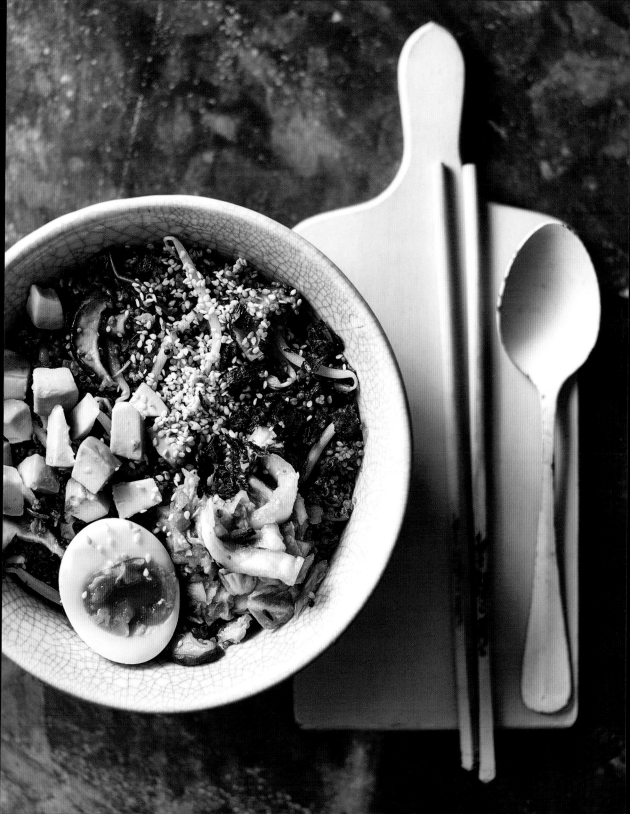

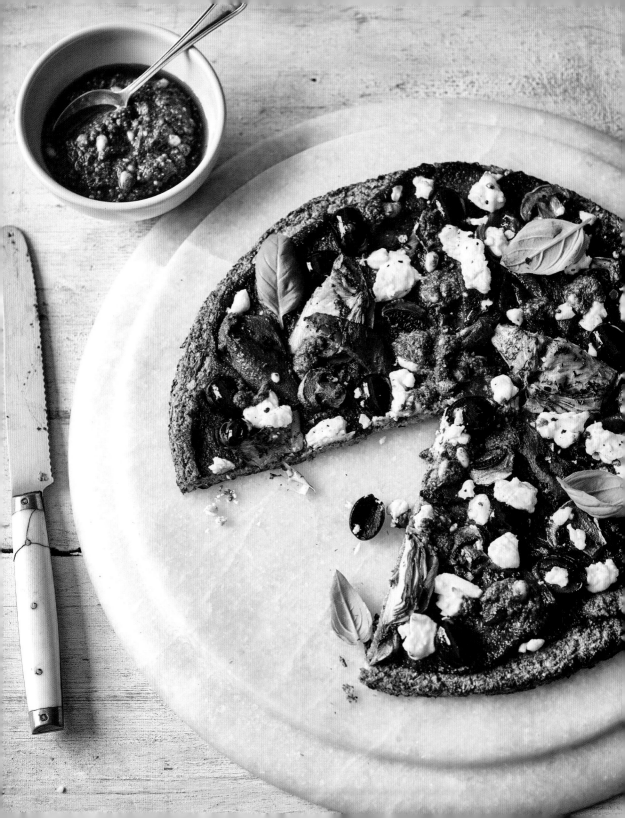

NUTRITIONAL INFORMATION PER SERVING 356 Kcals, **Protein** 35.8g,
**Carbohydrates** 18.2g of which sugars 14.3g, **Fat** 13.1 g of which saturates 6.3g

# Broccoli Pizza

There are many recipes out there for cauliflower pizza, but this alternative uses cauliflower and broccoli for the base, which gives the pizza a vibrant colour. To avoid dairy, omit the goat's cheese and add 3 tablespoons nutritional yeast flakes instead. Use your favourite toppings for your pizza.

Serves 2
Preparation: 20 minutes
Cooking: 30 minutes, plus
   5 minutes resting

olive oil, for greasing
1 head of broccoli, cut into florets
½ cauliflower, cut into florets
2 eggs
50g/1¾oz firm goat's cheese, grated
1 tsp garlic salt
1 tsp dried mixed herbs or oregano
ground black pepper
Pesto (pages 152–3), Ketchup
   (page 70), Fruity Barbecue Sauce
   (page 71) or tomato purée/paste

FOR THE TOPPING
Choose your favourites from:
  leftover roasted or steamed veg
    vegetables
  sliced mushrooms, tomatoes or
    red onions
  halved black olives
  sliced canned artichoke hearts
  thinly sliced deseeded red pepper/
    bell peppers
  cooked shellfish
  strips of cooked chicken

**1** Preheat the oven to 200°C/400°F/Gas 6. Grease a baking sheet with oil, then line it with baking parchment and grease the paper liberally.

**2** Put the broccoli and cauliflower florets into a food processor, or electric chopper, and pulse to form rice-like grains. Lightly steam the vegetable rice for 1 minute, or microwave for 2 minutes, then tip it into a clean dish towel or muslin cloth/cheesecloth. Allow it to cool slightly, then squeeze out as much excess liquid as possible.

**3** Put the rice back into the food processor and add the eggs, cheese, garlic salt and mixed herbs. Season with pepper, then pulse to combine.

**4** Spoon the mixture onto the prepared baking sheet, then use your hands to shape it to form a circle or rectangle, pressing down lightly and ensuring the edges all come together and there are no holes in the base. It should be about 2cm/¾in thick. Cook in the oven for 20 minutes or until golden and crisp.

**5** Spread with pesto or your chosen sauce and arrange your toppings of choice on top. Put back in the oven to heat through for 5–10 minutes. Leave to rest for 5 minutes, then slice and serve.

### Brain Benefits
Goat's cheese is a good source of vitamins D, A and K and B-vitamins, and is also high in tyrosine, an amino acid your body uses to produce the neurotransmitters that help alertness, concentration and motivation.

**V** NUTRITIONAL INFORMATION PER SERVING 318 Kcals, **Protein** 20.8g, **Carbohydrates** 20.9g of which sugars 14.4g, **Fat** 14g of which saturates 5.9g

# Cauliflower Egg Fried Rice

Crunchy cauliflower is a great substitute for rice: it is lower in carbs, but full of flavour. Ricing is an easy and tasty way to eat more cruciferous vegetables, which are important for detoxification as well as providing anti-inflammatory and antioxidant support. The protein in this dish comes from the eggs and edamame beans, making this an energizing meat-free option. Bags of frozen veggies are useful for getting meals together, making this a handy and speedy weekday meal. Leftovers can also be served cold for lunch the next day.

**Serves 2**
**Preparation: 15 minutes**
**Cooking: 12 minutes**

½ cauliflower
1 tbsp coconut oil or olive oil
2 eggs, lightly beaten
2 garlic cloves, crushed
3 spring onions/scallions, sliced
1 carrot, grated
½ red pepper/bell pepper,
    deseeded and diced
100g/3½oz/scant 1 cup frozen peas
100g/3½oz/¾ cup frozen shelled
    soy beans/edamame beans
1 tbsp tamari soy sauce
sea salt and ground black pepper
chopped coriander/cilantro leaves,
    to serve

**1** Put the cauliflower in a food processor, or electric chopper, and pulse until it resembles rice-like grains.

**2** Heat a little of the oil in a small frying pan over a medium heat. Add the eggs and cook as a flat omelette, it will take about 2 minutes to set.

**3** Remove the omelette from the pan and slice it into strips 2cm/¾in wide and leave to one side.

**4** Put the remaining oil in a large saucepan over a medium heat. Cook the garlic, spring onions/scallions, carrot and red pepper/bell pepper for 2 minutes, then add the peas and soy beans with a splash of water to prevent sticking. Cook for 5 minutes or until just tender.

**5** Add the cauliflower rice and the tamari. Stir to combine, then cover and cook for 3 minutes or until the cauliflower is just soft. Season with salt and pepper. Gently stir through the egg strips and scatter with coriander/cilantro to serve.

### Brain Benefits

Beans are a great source of B vitamins, particularly two neuro-protectors, folate and B6. These can help lower high homocysteine levels, which have been linked to cognitive decline and Alzheimer's.

# Sicilian Courgetti with Olives

Packed with healthy fats, thanks to the olives, and with plenty of antioxidant-rich herbs plus capers, this super-speedy meal is rich with flavour. Cannellini beans are delicious combined with tomatoes and roasted red peppers/bell peppers – a great storecupboard supper dish.

Serves 2
Preparation: 15 minutes
Cooking: 4–6 minutes, plus
   1–2 minutes standing

1 tbsp olive oil
125g/4½oz/¾ cup cherry tomatoes,
   cut in half
½ red onion, finely chopped
2 celery stalks, finely chopped
2 x 400g/14oz cans cannellini
   beans, drained and rinsed
60g/2¼oz/⅔ cup pitted black
   olives, cut in half
150g/5½oz/1 large roasted red
   pepper/bell pepper from a jar,
   drained and cut into strips
2 courgettes/zucchini, spiralized
sea salt and ground black pepper

FOR THE DRESSING
2 tbsp capers, drained and rinsed
1 garlic clove, crushed
1 handful of mint leaves
1 handful of coriander/cilantro leaves
1 handful of parsley leaves
2 tbsp flaxseed oil
3 tbsp extra virgin olive oil
3 tbsp red wine vinegar

**1** To make the dressing, put all the ingredients into a blender or food processor and whiz to combine. (This can be made ahead and stored in the refrigerator for 2–3 days.)

**2** Heat the oil in a large frying pan over a medium heat. Add the tomatoes, onion and celery, and cook for 3–4 minutes until the onion is soft. Tip in the beans, olives and red pepper/bell pepper. Season with salt and pepper, and heat through for 1–2 minutes.

**3** Add the courgettes/zucchini and mix well. Turn off the heat, then pour over the dressing and toss to combine. Allow the vegetables to stand for 1–2 minutes before serving to allow the courgette/zucchini to soak up the flavours. Serve.

**Brain Benefits**
Courgettes/zucchini are rich in immune-supporting vitamin C, and potassium, which helps to regulate blood pressure. The soluble fibre in the skin benefits the digestion and contributes towards healthy blood sugar levels.

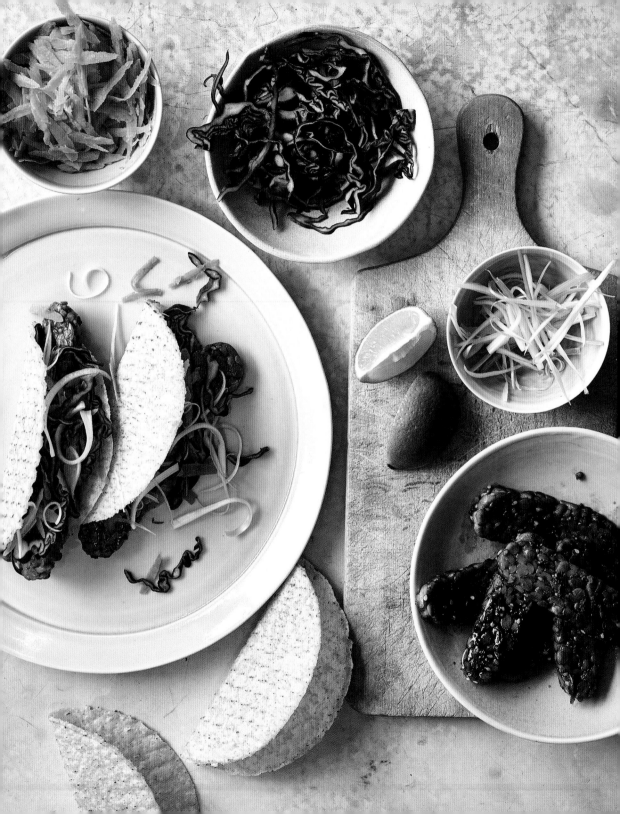

V  VE  NUTRITIONAL INFORMATION PER SERVING 385 Kcals, **Protein** 23.4g, **Carbohydrates** 33.5g of which sugars 14.2g, **Fat** 14.8g of which saturates 4.6g

# Sticky Orange Tempeh Tacos

Combined with sweet orange juice and spices, tempeh makes a perfect vegan protein-packed filling for corn tacos. It's a comforting, flavourful and healthy plant-based meal. You could also use firm tofu or a can of cooked cannellini beans instead of the tempeh.

Serves 2
Preparation: 15 minutes
Cooking: 7–8 minutes

1 tbsp coconut oil or olive oil
200g/7oz tempeh, cut into
    2cm/¾in slices
1 tsp sesame oil
3 tbsp tamari soy sauce
juice of 1 orange
½ tsp Chinese five-spice powder
5mm/¼in piece of root ginger,
    peeled and grated
1 garlic clove, crushed
2 tbsp yacon syrup
1 tsp sesame seeds
4 gluten-free corn taco shells
2 spring onions/scallions, chopped
1 carrot, grated
¼ red cabbage or lettuce, finely
    shredded
lime wedges and salad, to serve

**1** Heat the coconut oil in a frying pan and pan-fry the tempeh with a splash of water for 3–4 minutes until golden brown. Meanwhile, put the sesame oil in a bowl and add the tamari, orange juice, five-spice powder, ginger, garlic and yacon syrup. Combine well, then put to one side.

**2** Once the tempeh is golden brown, pour the tamari mixture into the pan and combine, then reduce the heat and cook for 2 minutes, to allow the sauce to reduce a little. Stir in the sesame seeds and remove from the heat.

**3** Heat the corn tacos for 2 minutes or according to the package directions. Fill each taco with the spring onions/scallions, carrot and cabbage, top with the tempeh and drizzle over the remaining sauce. Accompany with lime wedges and a salad.

### Brain Benefits

Tempeh is a fermented soy bean that originated in Indonesia and is a useful probiotic-rich food. It is a complete protein source and particularly high in B vitamins and zinc, which support cognitive function. It also contains vitamin K, which might help to reduce the risk of Alzheimer's disease, and magnesium to help calm the mind.

**V** **VE** NUTRITIONAL INFORMATION PER SERVING 500 Kcals, **Protein** 24g, **Carbohydrates** 56g of which sugars 4.2g, **Fat** 17.3g of which saturates 2.3g

# Mushroom Buddha Bowl with Miso Gravy

This recipe uses a mixture of button and portobello mushrooms, which have a wonderful meaty texture when roasted.

Serves 2
Preparation: 20 minutes, plus
    15 minutes soaking
Cooking: 40 minutes

80g wild rice or red rice or a
    mixture, rinsed
5g/⅛oz/¼ cup dried mushrooms
30g/1oz/¼ cup mixed seeds
1 tbsp mirin
150ml/5fl oz/⅔ cup vegetable stock
1 tbsp cornflour/cornstarch
1 tbsp white miso paste

FOR THE ROASTED MUSHROOMS
2 large portobello mushrooms,
    washed, stemmed, cut into
    2cm/¾in pieces (200g/7oz)
60g/2¼oz button mushrooms,
    thickly sliced
1 tbsp olive oil, plus extra for
    drizzling
2 tbsp balsamic vinegar
2 tbsp tamari soy sauce
100g/3½oz kale, shredded
400g/14oz can chickpeas, drained
    and rinsed

**1** Put the rice in a pan, cover with water and bring to the boil over a high heat, then reduce the heat and simmer for 40 minutes or until tender, or according to the package directions. Drain in a colander and keep warm.

**2** Meanwhile, put the dried mushrooms in a bowl and add 100ml/3½fl oz/scant ½ cup hot water. Leave to soak for 15 minutes, then strain through a sieve/fine-mesh strainer into a bowl, reserving the liquid. Put the seeds in a small saucepan and toast them over a medium-high heat for 30 seconds or until evenly toasted, shaking the pan frequently. Tip out of the pan onto a plate.

**3** Finely chop the mushrooms, then put them in a saucepan with the mirin and vegetable stock. Bring to the boil, then reduce the heat and simmer for 2 minutes. Put the cornflour/cornstarch in a small bowl and gradually stir in the mushroom liquid to form a smooth paste. Pour into the pan and cook for 2 minutes until it thickens, stirring constantly. Beat in the miso. Turn off the heat. Preheat the oven to 200°C/400°F/Gas 6.

**4** To make the roasted mushrooms, put the mushrooms in a bowl and toss in the oil, vinegar and tamari. Put on a baking sheet. Cook in the oven for 10 minutes or until just turning golden.

**5** Put the kale and chickpeas in a bowl and drizzle with olive oil. Add the kale and chickpeas to the mushrooms and return to the oven for 10 minutes or until the kale begins to crisp. Serve the rice with the mushroom and kale mixture, and the gravy, scattered with the seeds.

**V** **VE** NUTRITIONAL INFORMATION PER SERVING 305 Kcals, **Protein** 13.2g, **Carbohydrates** 31.6g of which sugars 6g, **Fat** 12.2g of which saturates 1.5g

# Cauliflower & Broccoli Butternut "Cheese"

This is a lovely vegan comfort dish. Using butternut squash and nutritional yeast flakes creates a delicious rich vegan version of a cheese sauce, which is tossed with veggies and topped with oats, then baked until crisp. For additional protein, you could toss in a can of cooked chickpeas.

**Serves 4**
**Preparation: 20 minutes**
**Cooking: 1 hour**

300g/10½oz butternut squash, peeled, deseeded and cut into chunks
2 tbsp olive oil
1 tbsp cornflour/cornstarch
200ml/7fl oz/scant 1 cup almond milk
6 tbsp nutritional yeast flakes
½ tsp ground turmeric
1 tsp Dijon mustard
½ tsp garlic powder
½ tsp onion powder
2 tsp fresh lemon juice
½ cauliflower, broken into florets
½ head of broccoli, broken into florets
100g/3½oz/1 cup gluten-free oats
30g/1oz/⅓ cup flaked/sliced almonds
sea salt and ground black pepper

**1** Preheat the oven to 190°C/375°F/Gas 5. Put the butternut squash on a baking sheet and drizzle with 1 tablespoon of the oil. Stir to coat, then season with salt and pepper. Cook in the oven for 30 minutes or until soft and lightly golden. Leave to cool.

**2** Put the cornflour/cornstarch in a bowl and mix with a little of the milk to make a smooth paste. Put the remaining milk in a saucepan and whisk in the cornflour paste followed by the nutritional yeast, turmeric, mustard, garlic powder, onion powder and lemon juice. Stir this sauce over a low heat for 5 minutes or until the mixture has thickened.

**3** Put the butternut squash and the sauce into a blender or food processor and whiz until thick and creamy. Adjust the seasoning.

**4** Bring a saucepan of water to the boil and add the cauliflower and broccoli. Cook for 3 minutes or until slightly softened. Drain in a colander and tip into an ovenproof dish. Pour over the sauce and stir in. In a bowl, mix the oats with the almonds and the remaining oil, then scatter over the dish. Cook in the oven for 20 minutes or until the top is golden, then serve.

**Brain Benefits**
Butternut squash is rich in carotenoids, while cauliflower and broccoli contain glucosinolates, which help to eliminate toxins, thereby reducing potential free-radical damage to cells, including brain cells.

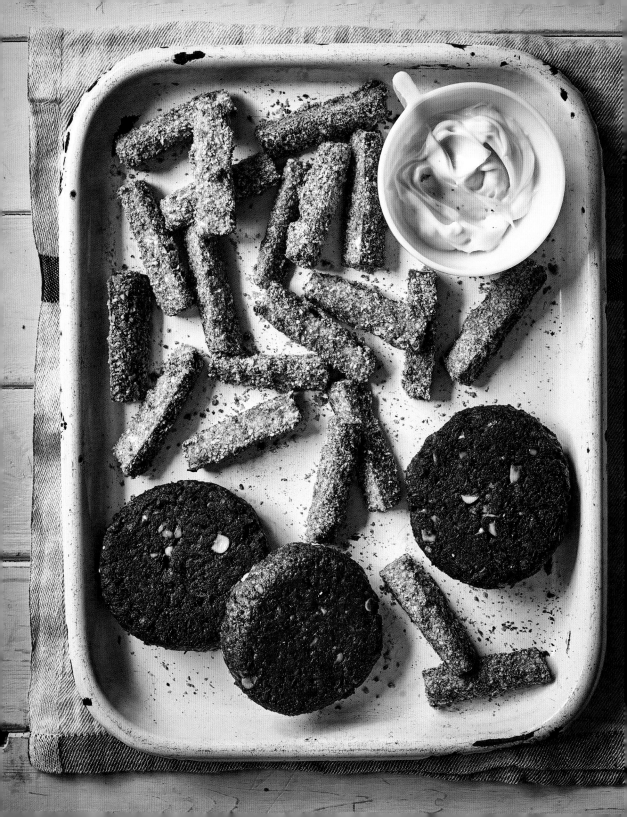

# Mexican Bean Burgers & Courgette Fries

**These vegetarian burgers have a delicious smoky chipotle flavour. Adding beans provides plenty of protein and you can use red kidney beans instead of the black beans, if you prefer.**

Serves 4
Preparation: 30 minutes, plus
   30 minutes soaking
Cooking: 15 minutes

½ dried chipotle chilli
olive oil, for greasing
2 garlic cloves, chopped
½ small onion, chopped
2 tbsp tamari soy sauce
3 tbsp tomato purée/paste
½ tsp ground cumin
½ tsp ground coriander
400g/14oz can black beans, drained
   and rinsed
80g/2¾oz/¾ cup gluten-free oats
1 tbsp ground flaxseed
60g/2¼oz canned sweetcorn,
   drained
sea salt and ground black pepper

FOR THE FRIES
60g/2¼oz/scant ⅔ cup ground
   almonds
2 tsp smoked paprika
2 tbsp nutritional yeast flakes
1 egg
1 large courgette/zucchini, cut
   lengthways into thick fingers

**1** Soak the chipotle chilli in water for 30 minutes, then drain. Preheat the oven to 200°C/400°F/Gas 6 and line two baking sheets with baking parchment, then grease the paper on one of them.

**2** Put the chipotle in a food processor and add the garlic, onion, tamari, tomato purée/paste and spices, then whiz to form a thick paste. Add the beans, oats, flaxseed and sweetcorn. Season with salt and pepper, and whiz briefly to combine everything, retaining some texture. Divide the mixture into four, then wet your hands and shape into burgers. (The burgers can now be frozen for up to 3 months, if you like.) Leave to one side.

**3** Preheat the grill/broiler to medium. Put the burgers on the greased baking sheet, then grill/broil for 5 minutes on each side until golden and crisp. (If you are cooking from frozen, bake at 200°C/400°F/Gas 6 for 20–30 minutes until cooked through and lightly browned.)

**4** Meanwhile, to make the fries, put the almonds in a wide, shallow dish and add the paprika and yeast flakes. Put the egg in a shallow bowl and beat it with a pinch of salt. Dip each courgette/zucchini finger in egg and then in the crumb mixture, coating well. Arrange the fries on the ungreased baking sheet and bake for 15 minutes or until golden and crispy. Serve the burgers with the fries.

### Brain Benefits
These protein-rich vegetarian burgers have plenty of magnesium to help calm the mind, and plant antioxidants and vitamin E to protect brain cells from oxidative stress.

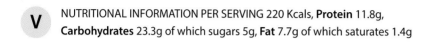

**V** NUTRITIONAL INFORMATION PER SERVING 220 Kcals, **Protein** 11.8g,
Carbohydrates 23.3g of which sugars 5g, **Fat** 7.7g of which saturates 1.4g

# Roasted Veggie Loaf

This loaf is a perfect way to use up leftover vegetables in the refrigerator; sweet potato, butternut squash and carrot, or other root veg are particularly good. Topped with barbecue sauce, this is perfect served hot or cold.

Serves 6
Preparation: 20 minutes, plus
    making the barbecue sauce
Cooking: 2 hours

1 onion, cut into chunks
4 garlic cloves, peeled and left
    whole
200g/7oz butternut squash, peeled,
    deseeded and cut into chunks
4 celery stalks, cut into chunks
100g/3½oz/2 cups broccoli florets
1 tbsp olive oil, plus extra for
    greasing
100g/3½oz/heaping ½ cup dried
    split peas
3 eggs
30g/1oz/¼ cup mixed seeds
60g/2¼oz/heaping ½ cup gluten-
    free oats
300g/10½oz Fruity Barbecue Sauce
    (page 71), or Ketchup (page 70)
    or passata
sea salt and ground black pepper

1 Preheat the oven 200°C/400°F/Gas 6 and grease and base-line a 900g/2lb loaf pan with baking parchment. Put the onion on a baking sheet and add the garlic, butternut squash, celery and broccoli. Drizzle with the olive oil and season with salt and pepper. Roast in the oven for 30 minutes or until just tender. Remove from the oven and leave to cool. Reduce the oven temperature to 160°C/315°F/Gas 2½.

2 Meanwhile, put the split peas in a saucepan of boiling water over a high heat. Bring to the boil, then reduce the heat and simmer for 30 minutes or until tender. Drain well.

3 Put the roasted vegetables in a food processor, or electric chopper, and pulse until they resemble breadcrumbs. Add the eggs and split peas, and pulse to combine. Stir in the seeds and the oats, and pulse again to combine, retaining some texture. Spoon into the lined loaf pan and press down the top firmly. Spoon over the barbecue sauce.

4 Cover the pan with foil, then bake for 1½ hours or until a skewer inserted into the centre of the loaf comes out clean. Leave to cool in the pan for 10 minutes, then remove and cut into thick slices. Serve warm or cold.

### Brain Benefits
Split peas are a good source of protein and gut-healthy fibre. They also contain plenty of B vitamins and the amino acid, tryptophan, needed to manufacture the neurotransmitter, serotonin, which regulates mood, appetite, hunger and sleep.

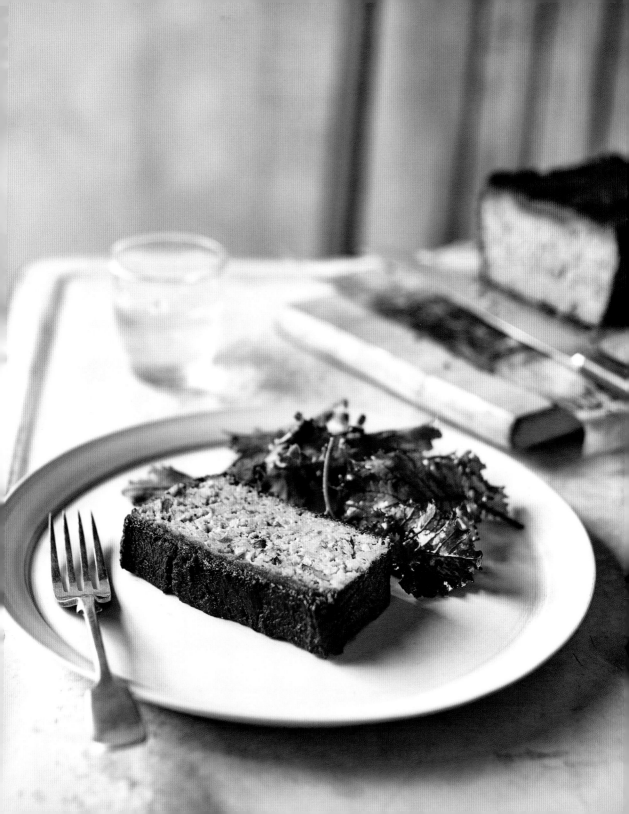

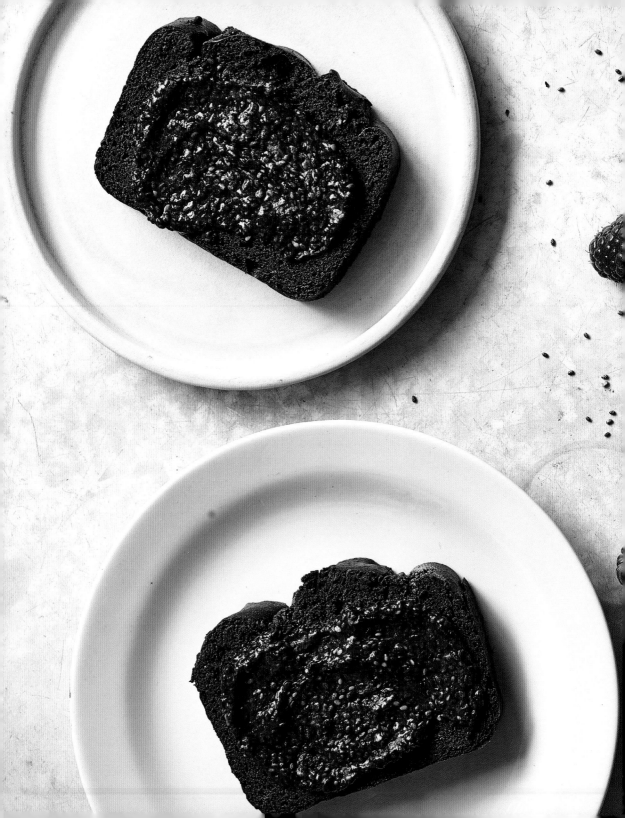

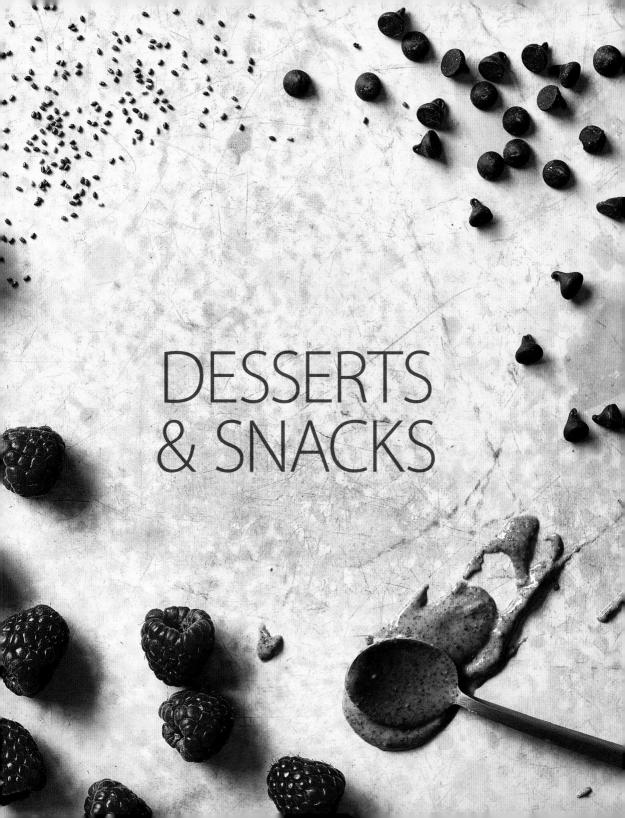

# DESSERTS & SNACKS

# Lemon Cheesecake Layered Pots

**Creamy and simple to make, these delicious tangy desserts would also be ideal as a breakfast option. They are rich, so a little goes a long way. You could use Granola (page 88) instead of the crumble in this recipe, if you prefer.**

Serves 4
Preparation: 20 minutes, plus
   30 minutes chilling

1 ripe avocado, pitted and skinned
zest and juice of 1 lemon
60g/2¼oz cacao butter or coconut
   oil
60g/2¼oz/⅓ cup xylitol or
   erythritol, or granulated stevia,
   to taste
100g/3½oz coconut yogurt or thick
   Greek yogurt, plus 2 tbsp for
   topping (optional)

FOR THE CRUMBLE
30g/1oz/scant ¼ cup walnuts,
   roughly chopped
30g/1oz/⅓ cup pecan nuts, roughly
   chopped
40g/1½oz/scant ½ cup gluten-free
   oats
1 tbsp desiccated/dried shredded
   coconut
juice of ½ lemon
1 tbsp xylitol or erythritol, or 2 tsp
   granulated stevia

**1** To make the crumble, put all the ingredients in a food processor, or electric chopper, and whiz to form chunky crumbs. Tip into a bowl and leave to one side.

**2** Put the avocado in the cleaned food processor or a blender and add the lemon zest and juice, the cacao butter, xylitol and yogurt, and whiz until smooth. Adjust the sweetness, to taste.

**3** Spoon a little of the crumble mixture into the base of four glasses. Top with avocado mixture, then more crumble. Reserve a little of the crumble mixture for sprinkling over the top. You can also top with a little coconut yogurt, if you like. Put in the refrigerator for 30 minutes to firm up slightly before serving.

Brain Benefits

The avocado in this dish is an excellent source of healthy brain-supporting fats. B vitamins are also present and are used by the body for the production of neurotransmitters for brain health.

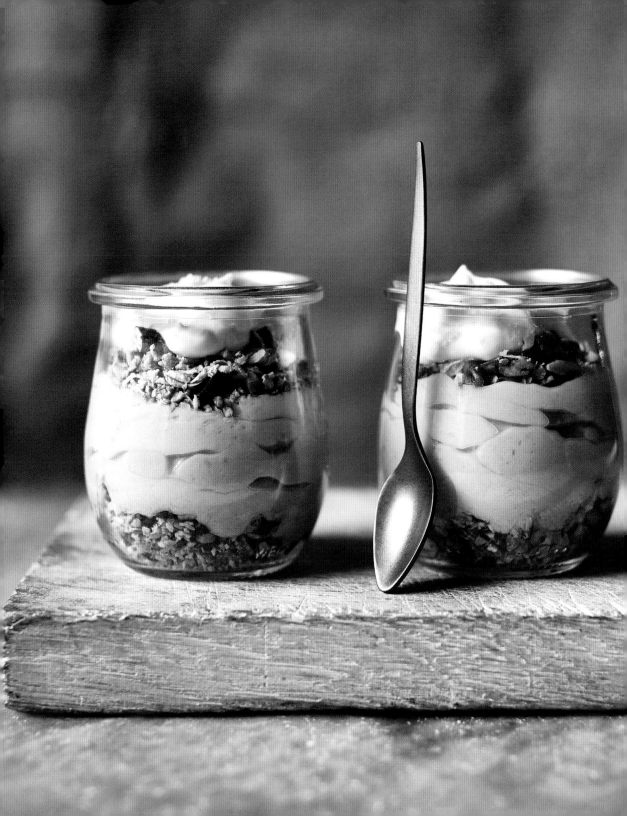

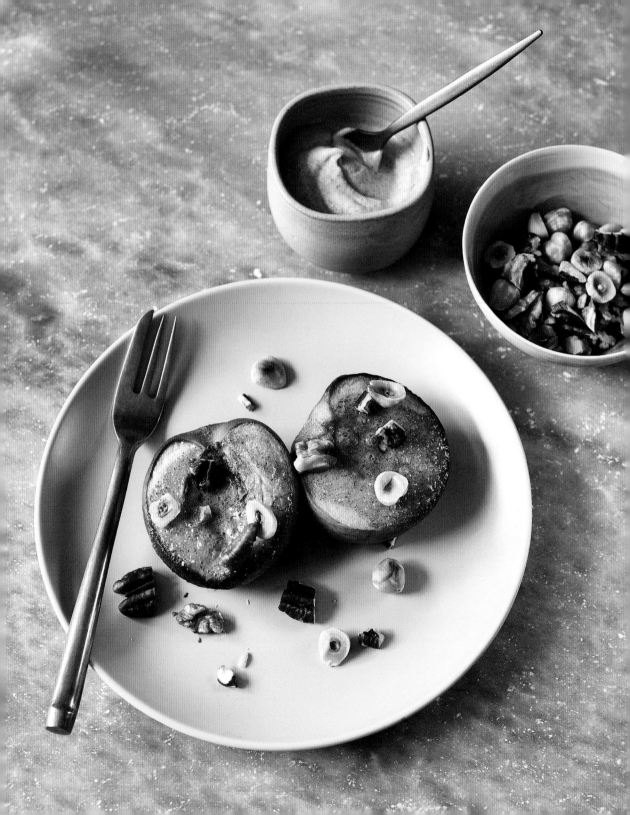

# Cinnamon Cream Peaches

**Light and simple, this summery dessert is perfect served warm or cold. You could also scatter over toasted nuts or homemade granola and serve with additional coconut yogurt, if you like. For a dairy-free version, use the coconut oil.**

Serves 2
Preparation: 15 minutes
Cooking: 20 minutes

2 peaches, cut in half and pitted
2 tbsp coconut oil or butter, melted
4 tbsp cream from the top of a can
    of full-fat coconut milk
1 tsp ground cinnamon
1 tsp vanilla extract
1 tbsp yacon syrup or rice malt
    syrup
ground cinnamon, for dusting
toasted nuts or Granola (page 88)
    (optional), to decorate

**1** Preheat the oven to 180°C/350°F/Gas 4 and line a baking sheet with baking parchment. Dip each peach half in the melted oil and put, cut-side up, on the prepared baking sheet.

**2** Put the coconut cream in a bowl and add the cinnamon, vanilla and yacon syrup. Beat together with a whisk or hand-held/immersion blender or food processor until creamy. Spoon the mixture into the middle of the peaches.

**3** Bake for 20 minutes or until the tops are light and golden. Serve with a dusting of cinnamon, and scatter over toasted nuts or granola, if you like.

### Brain Benefits

Peaches have strong antioxidant and anti-inflammatory properties, which help to protect the body from the effects of free-radicals. The fruit is also rich in soluble fibre, which is traditionally used to treat constipation and diarrhoea.

NUTRITIONAL INFORMATION PER SERVING 136 Kcals, **Protein** 2.4g, **Carbohydrates** 19.7g of which sugars 4.7g, **Fat** 4.8g of which saturates 4.1g

# Matcha Coconut Ice Cream

Here is a quick-to-prepare ice cream that also has a health boost from anti-inflammatory matcha green tea. I like to use a little MCT oil in this recipe for a brain boost, but if this is not available, simply omit it from the recipe. Adding lemon juice helps to balance the strong matcha flavour, and using xylitol keeps the sugar content low.

Serves 4

Preparation: 5 minutes, plus
    4–6 hours freezing

400ml/14fl oz can full-fat coconut
    milk
2–3 tsp matcha green tea powder,
    to taste
1 tsp vanilla extract
¼ tsp xanthan gum (optional)
2 tbsp coconut oil, softened
1 tbsp MCT oil (optional)
1 tbsp lemon juice
60g/2¼oz/⅓ cup xylitol, or
    erythritol, or granulated stevia,
    to taste

**1** Put all the ingredients in a high-speed blender or food processor and whiz until smooth and creamy. Using an ice-cream maker, churn the ice cream according to the manufacturer's directions.

**2** Either serve immediately or transfer to a freezerproof container and freeze until needed. (Alternatively, pour the mixture into a shallow, freezerproof container and freeze for 2 hours, then stir with a fork or use an electric hand whisk/beater, to break up the ice crystals, then freeze again for another 1–2 hours. Stir again and freeze for 1–2 hours until set.) The ice cream can be stored in the freezer for up to 3 months. Remove from the freezer 20 minutes before serving to allow it to soften slightly.

### Brain Benefits

Matcha green tea is packed with polyphenols, including epigallocatechin-3-gallate (EGCG), one of the most powerful catechins known for its potent anti-inflammatory benefits. Matcha powdered green tea has at least 100 times more antioxidants than regularly brewed green tea, meaning that even a small amount can give you significant benefits.

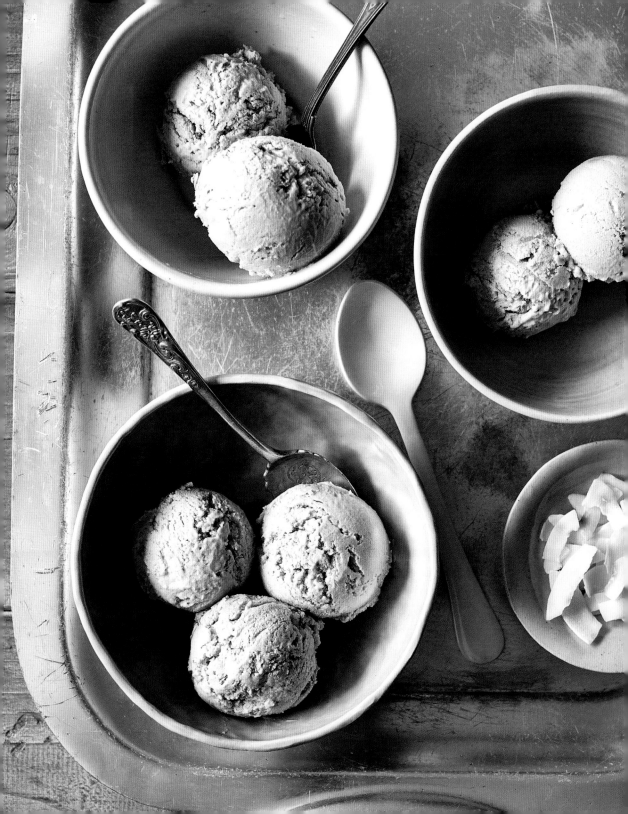

# Protein-Boost Mug Cakes

Mug cakes are easy, speedy treats made for one. All they take is a quick mix of the ingredients in a mug that you then microwave for a couple of minutes. In no time you can create a delicious, fluffy, moist cake that is perfect as a sweet treat, a pick-me-up snack or even a breakfast option. If you don't have a microwave, you can simply bake them for a little longer in the oven.

*They are perfect as a sweet treat, a pick-me-up snack or even breakfast.*

## Maca & Cinnamon-Spiced Protein Mug Cake

**V** NUTRITIONAL INFORMATION PER SERVING 313 Kcals, **Protein** 35g, **Carbohydrates** 19.4g of which sugars 0.7g, **Fat** 9.1g of which saturates 3.4g

SERVES 1  PREPARATION: 5 minutes  COOKING: 2 minutes (microwave)/15 minutes (oven), plus 5 minutes cooling

÷ coconut oil, for greasing ÷30g/1oz/scant ¼ cup vanilla protein powder ÷½ tsp baking powder ÷1 tbsp coconut flour ÷1 tsp maca powder ÷½ tsp ground cinnamon ÷1 tbsp xylitol or erythritol, or granulated stevia ÷1 large egg ÷4 tbsp almond milk ÷½ tsp vanilla extract ÷½ tsp ground cinnamon ÷1 tbsp yogurt

**1** If cooking in an oven, preheat the oven to 180°C/350°F/Gas 4 and lightly grease a microwaveable/ovenproof mug with a little oil.

**2** Put all the ingredients, except the cinnamon and yogurt, in the prepared mug and beat well with a fork to form a thick batter. Microwave on full power for 1–2 minutes or bake for 15 minutes or until firm to the touch. Leave to cool for 5 minutes.

**3** Mix together the cinnamon and yogurt. Serve the cake with a dollop of the yogurt.

# VARIATIONS

## ➤ VEGAN CHOCOLATE PEANUT BUTTER

✢ 3 tbsp ground almonds ✢ 30g/1oz/scant ¼ cup chocolate protein powder ✢ ½ tsp baking powder ✢ 4 tbsp almond milk ✢ 2 tsp peanut butter or other nut butter ✢ 2 tbsp apple sauce ✢ 1 tsp xylitol (optional) ✢ 1 small square of dark/bittersweet chocolate ✢ 1 tbsp yogurt

Put the almonds into the prepared mug followed by all the other ingredients, except the chocolate and yogurt, ending by pushing the square of chocolate down into the middle of the mixture. Cook as opposite and serve with the yogurt.

## ➤ MOCHA BREAKFAST CAKE

✢ 1 tsp raw cacao powder ✢ 30g/1oz/scant ¼ cup chocolate protein powder ✢ 1 tsp espresso coffee ✢ ½ tsp baking powder ✢ 1 tbsp coconut yogurt ✢ 1 tsp xylitol or erythritol ✢ 1 large egg ✢ 4 tbsp coconut cream or almond milk ✢ 1 drop of coffee extract (optional)

Put all the ingredients into the prepared mug. Beat well as opposite, adding a further 1 tablespoon coconut cream if needed to make a thick batter. Cook as opposite and serve with a drizzle of coconut cream or milk, if you like.

## ➤ BERRY CRUMBLE

✢ 2 tbsp Berry Chia Jam (see page 73) ✢ 30g/1oz/scant ¼ cup berry or vanilla protein powder ✢ 3 tbsp gluten-free plain flour or ground almonds ✢ ½ tsp baking powder ✢ 1 egg ✢ 2 tbsp almond milk ✢ 3 fresh raspberries ✢ 1 tbsp gluten-free oats or chopped nuts

Put the chia jam, protein powder, flour, baking powder, egg and almond milk into the prepred mug. Beat well as opposite, adding a further 1 tablespoon almond milk if needed to make a thick batter. Drop in the raspberries, then scatter the top with the oats or nuts and press in slightly. Cook as opposite and serve with yogurt and/or additional berry chia jam, if you like.

### Brain Benefits

These protein mug cakes make a delicious sweet treat, providing plenty of essential amino acids, choline from the eggs and healthy fats to support cognition.

**V** NUTRITIONAL INFORMATION PER SERVING 188 Kcals, **Protein** 4.9g, **Carbohydrates** 17.4g of which sugars 5.6g, **Fat** 10.7g of which saturates 4.5g

# Superberry Swirl Kefir Ice Cream

**Probiotic-rich kefir makes a wonderful ice cream combined with polyphenol-abundant berries and superberry powder. You can use coconut or milk kefir or yogurt for this recipe. For a Paleo or vegan version, use coconut kefir.**

Serves 6

Preparation: 15 minutes, plus
    making the kefir and 1 hour
    optional soaking and up to
    4 hours freezing

Cooking: 5 minutes

80g/2¾oz/⅔ cup cashew nuts

100g/3½oz/¾ cup fresh or frozen
    mixed berries

100g/3½oz/¾ cup fresh or frozen
    cherries, pitted

juice of ½ lemon

300ml/10½fl oz/scant 1⅓ cups Milk
    Kefir or Coconut Kefir (page 63)

1 tbsp vanilla extract

1 tsp acai berry powder or
    superberry powder (optional)

60g/2¼oz/⅓ cup xylitol or
    erythritol

2 tbsp coconut oil

a pinch of sea salt

**1** If you have time, soak the cashew nuts in water for 1 hour, then drain in a colander. Leave to one side. If using fresh fruit, put the fruit in a saucepan with the lemon juice and a splash of water, and simmer gently for 5 minutes or until soft.

**2** If using frozen fruit, allow the berries to defrost slightly. Put into a blender or food processor and whiz with the lemon juice to form a purée. Pour into a bowl or jug and leave to one side. Put the nuts in the cleaned blender and add the kefir, vanilla, acai berry powder, xylitol, oil and salt, then whiz until smooth and creamy.

**3** Pour the kefir mixture into an ice-cream maker and churn according to the manufacturer's directions; as it begins to thicken and freeze, slowly pour in the fruit purée and continue to churn. Serve immediately or transfer to a freezerproof container and freeze for up to 3 months. (Alternatively, pour the blended mixture, including the berry purée, into a shallow, freezerproof container and freeze for 2 hours, then stir with a fork or use an electric hand whisk/beater to break up the ice crystals, then freeze again for another 1–2 hours. Stir again and freeze for 1–2 hours until set.)

### Brain Benefits

Cherries are rich in fibre and protective antioxidants, vitamin C, carotenoids and anthocyanins. Cherries have also been shown to lower inflammation. Adding acai berry powder is an easy way to further increase this dessert's antioxidant benefits as well as providing trace minerals and B vitamins.

NUTRITIONAL INFORMATION PER MUFFIN 275 Kcals, **Protein** 9.6g, **Carbohydrates** 8.1g of which sugars 2.3g, **Fat** 22.2 g of which saturates 4.3g

# Orange Blueberry Muffins

These fabulously moist Paleo muffins are packed with antioxidant-rich blueberries. They also contain olive oil, which keeps them lovely and moist.

Makes 10 muffins
Preparation: 15 minutes
Cooking: 20 minutes

50ml/1¾fl oz/scant ¼ cup olive oil, plus extra for greasing
190g/6¾oz/scant 1 cup almond butter
80g/2¾oz/¾ cup ground almonds
3 eggs
50g/1¾oz/scant ⅓ cup xylitol or erythritol
zest of 1 orange
2 tbsp orange juice
2 tbsp desiccated/dried shredded coconut
½ tsp bicarbonate of soda/baking soda
1 tsp baking powder
a pinch of sea salt
¼ tsp ground cinnamon
90g/3¼oz/scant ¾ cup frozen blueberries

**1** Preheat the oven to 180°C/350°F/Gas 4 and grease a 10-cup muffin tray. Put all the ingredients, except the blueberries, into a food processor and whiz to form a smooth batter. Add the blueberries and pulse very briefly or simply stir them in to prevent breaking up the blueberries too much.

**2** Spoon the mixture into the prepared muffin cups. Bake for 20 minutes or until golden and cooked through and firm to the touch. Cool in the tray, then turn out to serve.

### Brain Benefits
Rich in healthy monounsaturated fats, olive oil is a staple of Mediterranean diets, known for their longevity-boosting properties and brain-supporting benefits. Oranges and blueberries provide plenty of vitamin C and antioxidants, which have been shown to stimulate the flow of blood and oxygen to the brain, thereby keeping the mind fresh.

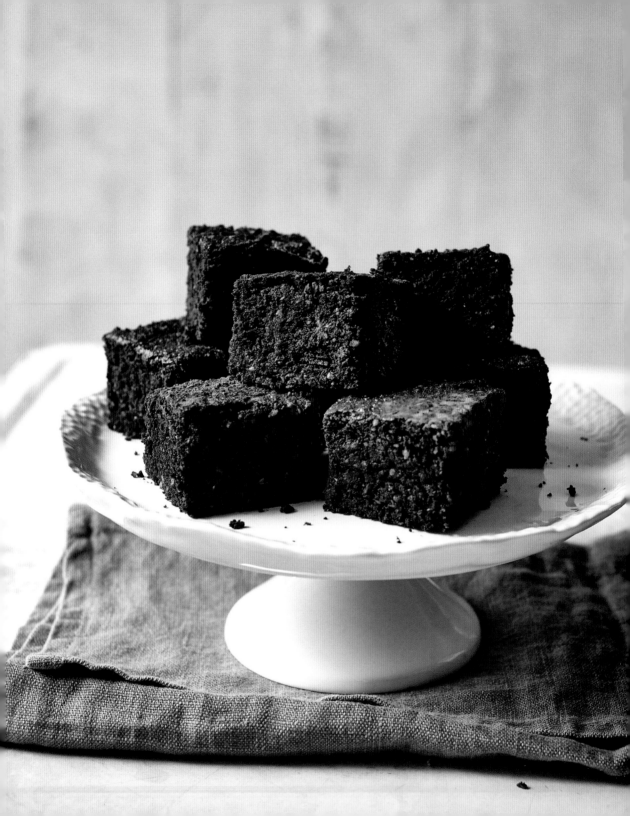

# Beet Chocolate Brownies

Rich and fudgy, these delicious beetroot/beet brownies are packed with protein, thanks to the addition of nut butter and protein powder. They are perfect as a healthy snack, breakfast on the go or a pick-me-up when energy levels are flagging.

Makes 16 brownies
Preparation: 15 minutes
Cooking: 20–25 minutes

olive oil, for greasing
2 cooked beetroots/beets
200g/7oz/scant 1 cup almond
    nut butter
200g/7oz dark/bittersweet
    chocolate, chopped
80g/2¾oz/scant ½ cup xylitol or
    erythritol
3 eggs
1 tsp vanilla extract
30g/1oz/scant ¼ cup chocolate or
    vanilla protein powder
60g/2¼oz/scant ⅔ cup ground
    almonds
1 tsp ground cinnamon
1 tsp bicarbonate of soda/baking
    soda
1 tsp baking powder
60g/2¼oz shelled hemp seeds

**1** Preheat the oven to 180°C/350°F/Gas 4 and grease and line a 20cm/8in square baking pan with baking parchment. Grate the beetroots/beets and leave to one side.

**2** Put the nut butter in a saucepan and add the chocolate and xylitol. Warm gently over a medium-low heat to melt the chocolate. Allow the chocolate to cool slightly. Put in a food processor and add the eggs, vanilla, protein powder, ground almonds, cinnamon, bicarbonate of soda/baking soda and baking powder, and whiz to combine. Whiz in the beetroots and hemp seeds.

**3** Spoon the mixture evenly into the prepared pan. Bake for 20–25 minutes until golden brown and firm to the touch. Leave to cool completely before removing from the tray. Cut into 16 squares. Store in the refrigerator for up to 5 days or freeze for up to 3 months.

**Brain Benefits**
Beetroot/beet is a fabulous brain-boosting food known to help the production of nitric oxide and improve vasodilation in the body and brain. The hemp seeds are a great source of additional protein and omega-3 fats.

**V**   NUTRITIONAL INFORMATION PER SLICE 394 Kcals, **Protein** 7.4g, **Carbohydrates** 25.6g of which sugars 2.2g, **Fat** 29.1g of which saturates 11.7g

# Green Lime Cream Cake

**Spinach is a surprising and healthy ingredient in this delicious gluten-free green cake. It is topped with a lime cream, but you could simply serve the cake with Greek yogurt or coconut yogurt, if you prefer.**

Makes 1 cake/10 slices
Preparation: 15 minutes, plus
    overnight chilling
Cooking: 40–50 minutes

200g/7oz/heaping ¾ cup butter
    or coconut oil, plus extra for
    greasing
100g/3½oz/heaping ½ cup xylitol
    or erythritol
3 eggs
1 tsp vanilla extract
zest of 2 limes
2 tbsp lime juice
40g spinach leaves
200g/7oz/2 cups ground almonds
100g/3½oz/⅔ cup fine polenta/
    cornmeal
1 tsp baking powder
½ tsp bicarbonate of soda/baking
    soda

FOR THE LIME CREAM
2 x 400ml/14fl oz cans full-fat
    coconut milk
juice of 1 lime
3 tbsp xylitol or erythritol, finely
    ground
lime zest and coconut flakes, to
    decorate

**1** Put the unopened cans of coconut milk for the lime cream upright in the refrigerator overnight – this allows the thick cream to harden at the top of the cans.

**2** The next day, preheat the oven to 160°C/315°F/Gas 2½/Gas 3 and grease and line a 20cm/8in springform cake pan with baking parchment.

**3** Put the butter in a food processor and add the xylitol, then whiz until light and creamy. Gradually beat in the eggs, vanilla and the lime zest and juice. Add the remaining ingredients and combine.

**4** Spoon the batter into the prepared cake pan. Bake for 40–50 minutes until the cake is golden and a skewer inserted into the centre comes out clean. Leave the cake to cool in the pan for 10 minutes, then turn out onto a wire rack to cool completely.

**5** To make the lime cream, open the cans of coconut milk and scoop out the thick cream from each one into a small bowl or jug/pitcher. (The liquid underneath can be used as a drink added to smoothies or curries. You can also freeze this liquid if you don't wish to use it immediately.) Add the lime juice and xylitol and, using a hand-held/immersion blender, beat together until creamy. Spread the coconut cream over the cake and decorate with lime zest and coconut flakes.

### Brain Benefits
Limes are a good source of vitamin C and antioxidants, including limonene, known for its detoxification and anti-inflammatory benefits.

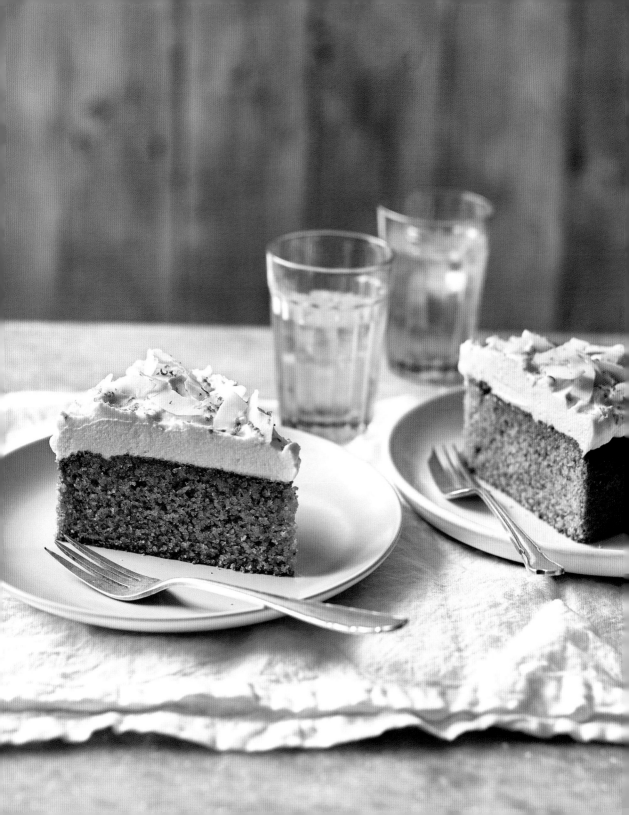

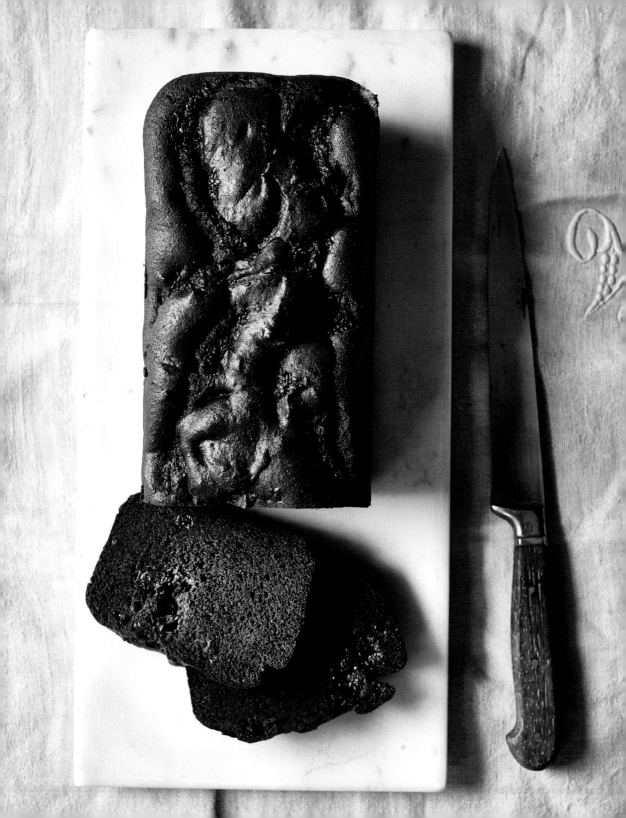

# Chocolate Berry Swirl Bread

Some of my Berry Chia Jam is swirled into this rich-tasting and moist bread to create a lovely crimson colour. Slice the loaf and spread with additional chia jam – it's delicious lightly toasted, too.

Makes 900g/2lb loaf/10 slices

Preparation: 15 minutes, plus
    making the jam

Cooking: 45 minutes

coconut oil, for greasing

2 ripe bananas

200g/7oz/scant 1 cup nut butter,
    such as almond, cashew nut,
    sunflower seed butter

50g/1¾oz/scant ⅓ cup xylitol or
    erythritol

3 eggs

30g/1oz/¼ cup unsweetened cocoa
    or raw cacao powder

30g/1oz/¼ cup coconut flour

½ tsp bicarbonate of soda/baking
    soda

1 tsp baking powder

½ tsp ground cinnamon

a pinch of sea salt

30g/1oz/scant ¼ cup chocolate
    chips

½ x quantity Berry Chia Jam (page
    73) or pure fruit spread

**1** Preheat the oven to 180°C/350°F/Gas 4 and grease and line a 900g/2lb loaf pan with baking parchment. Put all the ingredients, except the chocolate chips and chia jam, into a food processor and whiz to combine. (Alternatively, mash the bananas and put in a bowl. Mix together well with the above ingredients using an electric hand whisk/beater.) Stir in the chocolate chips.

**2** Pour the batter into the prepared loaf pan. Spoon the berry chia jam in a few separate spoonfuls over the top, then swirl it through the batter using a knife or spoon. Bake for 45 minutes or until firm and lightly browned on the top.

**3** Leave the bread to cool for 15 minutes in the pan before turning out onto a wire rack to cool completely. Store in the refrigerator, wrapped, for up to 1 week, or freeze for up to 3 months.

### Brain Benefits

Bananas and coconut flour provide plenty of prebiotic fibre to support gut health. Bananas are rich in tryptophan and tyrosine – amino acids that your body uses to make the neurotransmitters, serotonin and dopamine, which help to regulate your mood. Bananas are also rich in magnesium to help calm the mind and body, thereby improving sleep and relaxation.

P  V  NUTRITIONAL INFORMATION PER COOKIE SANDWICH 286 Kcals, **Protein** 11.1g, **Carbohydrates** 14.1g of which sugars 0.9g, **Fat** 20.2g of which saturates 7.2g

# Cinnamon Nut Butter Cookies

These cookies are high in protein, thanks to the addition of protein powder and almond flour. They are filled with a delicious nut butter here, but you could just as well eat the cookies on their own.

Makes 8 cookie sandwiches
Preparation: 20 minutes
Cooking: 15 minutes

130g/4¾oz/scant 1⅓ cups almond flour
30g/1oz arrowroot powder
20g/¾oz/scant ¼ cup raw cacao powder
30g/1oz/scant ¼ cup vanilla protein powder
50g/1¾oz/¼ cup coconut oil
2 eggs
1 tbsp ground cinnamon
1 tbsp maca powder
a pinch of sea salt
1 tsp vanilla extract
40g/1½oz/heaping ¼ cup xylitol or erythritol

FOR THE FILLING
125g/4½oz/½ cup cashew nut butter
1 tbsp raw cacao powder
1 tsp maca powder
1 tsp vanilla extract
40g/1½oz/heaping ¼ cup xylitol or erythritol, finely ground
a little almond milk, if needed

**1** Preheat the oven to 180°C/350°F/Gas 4 and line a baking sheet with baking parchment. Put the almond flour into a food processor and add the arrowroot, cacao and protein powder, then whiz to combine. (Or put the ingredients in a bowl and mix well.) Add the remaining ingredients to the food processor and whiz to form a slightly soft dough. (Alternatively, mix the ingredients together well using an electric hand whisk/beater.)

**2** Roll the dough between two pieces of cling film/plastic wrap until 2cm/¾in thick. Stamp out 16 rounds using a 6cm/2½in cookie cutter. Put on the prepared baking sheet and bake for 15 minutes or until lightly golden. Transfer to a wire rack to cool completely.

**3** To make the filling, put the nut butter in a bowl and add the cacao, maca, vanilla and xylitol. Mix well together. This can be stored in the refrigerator until needed. Add a dash of almond milk, if needed, to form a smooth paste.

**4** Spread 1 teaspoon of the filling onto one cookie and put another cookie on top to form a sandwich. Repeat to make seven more. Store in an airtight container or in the refrigerator for up to 1 week.

Brain Benefits

Maca root is an adaptogen – it helps the body adapt to daily stresses. It can improve energy and focus and has the ability to restore hormone balance and to elevate the feel-good endorphins. It also provides a number of essential minerals, including magnesium, zinc, copper, iron and selenium.

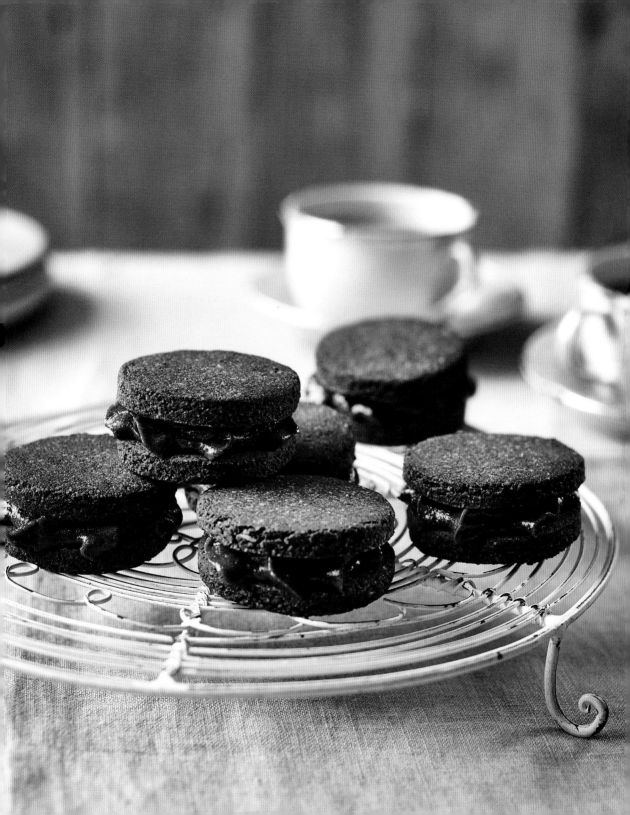

# Brain Protein Bliss Balls

These tempting bliss balls are much lower in sugar than many traditional recipes and are packed with brain-healthy antioxidants. The combination of turmeric, goji and orange gives these a wonderful, vibrant colour while helping to lower inflammation in the body and protect the brain's neurons from damage. For an additional boost, I have added lion's mane mushroom powder; you can use any medicinal mushroom powder or leave it out if it is unavailable. If your protein powder is sweetened, you may not need the yacon syrup.

**Makes 25 balls**
**Preparation: 15 minutes**

20g/¾oz/¼ cup desiccated/dried
    shredded coconut
60g/2¼oz/½ cup vanilla protein
    powder
1 tbsp yacon syrup
a pinch of sea salt
60g/2¼oz/¼ cup cashew nut butter
1 small orange, peeled, or
    60g/2¼oz frozen mango chunks
¼ tsp ground turmeric or 5mm/¼in
    piece of turmeric root, peeled
    and grated
1 tbsp maca powder
1 tbsp lion's mane medicinal
    powder (optional)
60g/2¼oz/2 heaping cups puffed
    brown rice cereal (unsweetened)
30g/1oz/¼ cup dried goji berries

**1** Put all the ingredients, except the goji berries, in a food processor and whiz until the mixture starts to come together. Add the goji berries and continue to whiz to break up the berries slightly.

**2** Take spoonfuls of the mixture and roll into balls. Put on a tray or plate. Store in the refrigerator for up to 1 week.

### Brain Benefits

Studies suggest that goji berries might offer neuro-protective and anti-ageing benefits. They are exceptionally rich in phytochemicals, which are known to support immune health and to offer antioxidant protection. They also contain carotenoids, including beta-carotene and lycopene, important protective antioxidants in the brain.

**P** NUTRITIONAL INFORMATION PER GUMMY 35 Kcals, **Protein** 2.2g,
**Carbohydrates** 2.6g of which sugars 0.6g, **Fat** 1.6g of which saturates 1.4g

# Strawberry Cream Gummies

These are tasty, probiotic-rich, creamy, real-fruit gummies. Remember to add the yogurt once the gelatine liquid has cooled slightly to preserve its probiotic benefits. If you don't have yogurt to hand, you can use coconut cream and empty a couple of probiotic capsules into the mixture as well.

**Makes 15 gummies**
**Preparation: 15 minutes, plus**
    **5 minutes soaking and cooling**
    **and 1–2 hours setting**
**Cooking: 1–2 minutes**

4 tbsp gelatine powder
150g/5½oz fresh or frozen
    strawberries
2 tbsp xylitol or erythritol, or a few
    drops of stevia liquid, to taste
125g/4½oz coconut yogurt, or
    coconut cream with 2 capsules
    of probiotics (opened)

**1** Put 5 tablespoons cold water in a bowl and sprinkle over the gelatine, then stir in. Allow the gelatine to soak for 5 minutes.

**2** Put the fruit and xylitol into a blender or food processor and whiz until smooth. Put the fruit purée in a saucepan and heat over a medium heat for 1–2 minutes until it comes to a simmer.

**3** Add the gelatine mixture and stir well until the gelatine has dissolved. Leave to cool slightly, then add the coconut yogurt and use a blender to whiz the mixture until smooth.

**4** Pour the mixture into little moulds or ice cube trays, or divide between small ramekins. Put in the refrigerator for 1–2 hours until set. Turn out of the moulds. Store in the refrigerator for up to 1 week.

### Brain Benefits

The antioxidants found in strawberries help to protect and repair cells from damage that can speed up the ageing process and contribute to cognitive decline. A type of protein derived from collagen, gelatine is beneficial for preventing intestinal damage and improving the lining of the digestive tract, thereby preventing permeability and leaky gut (see page 20).

**V** **VE** NUTRITIONAL INFORMATION PER SERVING 96 Kcals, **Protein** 6g, **Carbohydrates** 13.1g of which sugars 3.1g, **Fat** 1.3g of which saturates 0.2g

# Smoky Cauliflower Bites

**Crispy on the outside and soft in the middle, these nibbles are simple to make and a healthy alternative to popcorn.**

Serves 4
Preparation: 15 minutes
Cooking: 40 minutes

60g/2¼oz/½ cup chickpea flour/
    gram flour
1 tsp smoked paprika
a pinch of cayenne pepper
1 tsp xylitol or erythritol
1 tsp garlic salt
¼ tsp Dijon mustard
1 cauliflower, cut into bite-size
    pieces
ground black pepper

**1** Preheat the oven to 200°C/400°F/Gas 6 and line a baking sheet with baking parchment. Put all the ingredients, except the cauliflower, in a bowl. Season with pepper. Gradually whisk in 100ml/3½fl oz/scant ½ cup warm water or enough to make a thick, smooth batter.

**2** Toss the cauliflower pieces in the chickpea batter, making sure to coat each piece completely, then put the battered cauliflower onto the prepared baking sheet in an even layer.

**3** Bake for 20 minutes, then flip over and return to the oven for a further 20 minutes or until the bites are golden and crispy. Remove from the oven and leave to cool for 10 minutes before serving.

### Brain Benefits
Cauliflower is a member of the cruciferous family known for its ability to enhance detoxification. Cauliflower is anti-inflammatory and antioxidant-rich, which can help to optimize brain health.

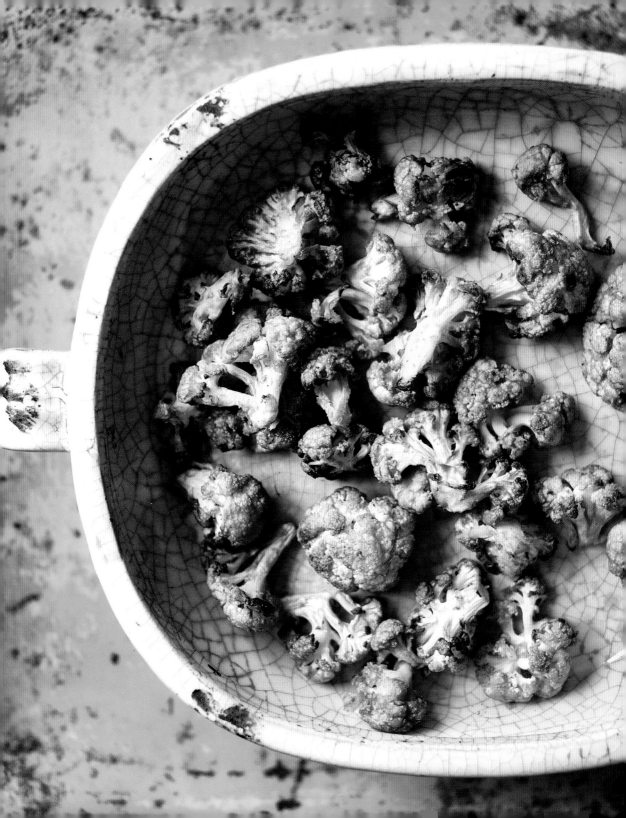

# Kale Crisps

Tasty kale crisps are one of my favourite go-to snacks. Packed with nutrients, antioxidants and fibre, they are healthy but by no means dull. There are plenty of ways to flavour them – you can even have sweet ones – so experiment with a range of flavours depending on what you have in your storecupboard. Use the same method as outlined below for each of these variations. The method below uses an oven. If you have a dehydrator, you will need to dehydrate them overnight at 7°C/45°F, then turn them over onto the mesh sheets and dehydrate for a further 6–8 hours until very crisp.

*Packed with nutrients, antioxidants and fibre, these crisps are healthy but by no means dull.*

## Kale Crisps

NUTRITIONAL INFORMATION PER SERVING 57 Kcals, **Protein** 2.5g,
**Carbohydrates** 2.9g of which sugars 1.9g, **Fat** 3.5g of which saturates 0.5g

ACCORDING TO CHOICES　SERVES 8 PREPARATION: 10 minutes, plus soaking where needed

COOKING: 30 minutes, plus 30 minutes drying

✛ **200g/7oz chopped kale leaves, large stems removed** ✛**flavourings as opposite**

**1** Preheat the oven to 110°C/225°F/Gas ¼ and line two baking sheets with baking parchment. Put the kale in a large bowl.
**2** Put your chosen flavouring ingredients into a blender or food processor and add about 100ml/3½fl oz/scant ½ cup water, or just enough to blend into a thick paste. Allow the mixture to stand for 1 minute, then whiz again (the addition of psyllium, chia or flaxseed in some recipes helps the mixture to thicken). Pour the mixture over the kale and, using your hands, massage the coating into the kale for a few minutes, making sure that all the kale pieces are fully coated.

**3** Tip the kale onto the prepared baking sheets and spread it out into a single layer. Cook in the oven for 30 minutes. Loosen the kale from the parchment using a spatula, then put the sheets back in the oven, turn the oven off, and leave them for 30 minutes or until the kale has crisped up. Store in an airtight container for up to 2 days.

# FLAVOURINGS

## ➤ SPICY TOMATO

The use of sun-dried tomato enhances the flavour of this coating. Using garlic salt is a quick way to give these crisps a delicious mild garlicky flavour, too.

✦ 60g/2¼oz/scant ½ cup sunflower seeds ✦ 3 tbsp nutritional yeast flakes ✦ 4 sun-dried tomatoes in oil, drained ✦ 1 tbsp apple cider vinegar ✦ 1 tsp garlic salt ✦ ½ tsp smoked paprika ✦ a pinch of dried chilli/hot pepper flakes (optional) ✦ 2 tbsp ground flaxseed

## ➤ CREAMY APPLE & CINNAMON

A lovely sweet crisp with plenty of warming cinnamon.

✦ 1 apple, chopped ✦ 1 tbsp vanilla extract ✦ 1 tbsp lemon juice ✦ 80g/2¾oz/⅔ cup cashew nuts (soaked for 1 hour, then drained) ✦ 2 tbsp xylitol or erythritol, or a little stevia, to taste ✦ 1 tbsp ground cinnamon ✦ a pinch of sea salt

## ➤ MACCACHINO

A lovely combination of maca and cacao powder combined with creamy tahini.

✦ 50g/1¾oz/½ cup raw cacao powder ✦ 1 tbsp maca powder ✦ 2 tbsp tahini ✦ 1–2 tbsp xylitol or erythritol, to taste ✦ 1 tbsp flaxseed ✦ a pinch of sea salt

## ➤ SWEET MISO VINEGAR

A tangy coating with a wonderful sweet-and-sour flavour.

✦ 1 tbsp white miso paste ✦ juice of 1 orange ✦ 2 tsp psyllium husks or 1 tbsp ground flaxseed ✦ 1 tbsp tamari soy sauce ✦ 2 tbsp rice vinegar ✦ 2 tbsp sesame seeds

## ➤ CHEESE & ONION

Turmeric gives the coating a lovely cheese-like colour and provides additional anti-inflammatory benefits, too.

✦ 125g/4½oz/1 cup cashew nuts or sunflower seeds (soaked for 1 hour, then drained) ✦ 1 red pepper/bell pepper, deseeded and chopped ✦ juice of 1 lemon ✦ 3 tbsp nutritional yeast flakes ✦ 1 tsp onion powder ✦ ½ tsp sea salt ✦ ¼ tsp ground turmeric

### Brain Benefits

Kale is a nutritional powerhouse, rich in phytochemicals including sulfurophane, which enhances liver detoxification, kaempferol and carotenoids to help lower inflammation. It also provides plant-based omega-3 ALA (alpha-linolenic acid) for overall brain function. The fibre in kale is beneficial for gut health.

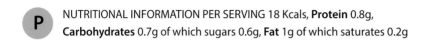

**P** NUTRITIONAL INFORMATION PER SERVING 18 Kcals, **Protein** 0.8g,
**Carbohydrates** 0.7g of which sugars 0.6g, **Fat** 1g of which saturates 0.2g

# Roasted Aubergine & Kale Tapenade

Traditional tapenade ingredients are combined with aubergine/eggplant and kale to boost the flavour and enhance its protective antioxidant properties. Serve this with vegetable sticks, spread on seeded crackers or toasted Paleo bread (see pages 211 and 94).

Serves 8
Preparation: 10 minutes
Cooking: 35 minutes

1 large aubergine/eggplant,
    cut into 2cm/¾in slices
4 garlic cloves, chopped
olive oil, for drizzling
1 tbsp apple cider vinegar
100g/3½oz kale, tough stalks
    removed, chopped
4 tbsp chopped parsley leaves
50g/1¾oz/½ cup pitted black olives
1 anchovy fillet in oil, drained
1 tbsp capers, drained and rinsed
sea salt

**1** Preheat the oven to 200°C/400°F/Gas 6. Season the aubergine/eggplant with a little salt, then put them on a baking sheet and add the garlic. Drizzle with olive oil and sprinkle over the vinegar, then roast in the oven for 30 minutes or until soft.

**2** Put the kale in a bowl and drizzle with olive oil, then mix well. Add to the baking sheet and roast for a further 5 minutes or until slightly crisp. Remove from the oven and leave to cool slightly.

**3** Put all the ingredients in a food processor and pulse until fairly smooth but retaining some texture. Store in the refrigerator for up to 1 week.

**Brain Benefits**
Aubergines/eggplants contain an antioxidant known as nasunin within the purple pigment of their skin. Researchers have reported that it helps to reduce free-radicals and may protect brain health.

**V** **VE** NUTRITIONAL INFORMATION PER SERVING 74 Kcals, **Protein** 3.2g, **Carbohydrates** 6.5g of which sugars 0.8g, **Fat** 3.4g of which saturates 0.4g

# Smashed Lemon Chickpea Spread

Preserved lemons give this spread a lovely tangy flavour. Use it as a dip with vegetable sticks or to spread on seed crackers or slices of my seeded bread (see pages 211 and 94).

Serves 6 as a spread/dip
Preparation: 10 minutes
Cooking: 3–4 minutes

2 tsp olive oil
½ onion, chopped
½ garlic clove, crushed
½ tsp ground cumin
½ tsp smoked paprika
4 pitted green olives, finely chopped
1 preserved lemon, flesh removed and rind finely chopped
1 tomato, finely chopped
400g/14oz can chickpeas, drained and rinsed
2 tsp tahini
sea salt and ground black pepper
chopped parsley leaves, to serve

**1** Heat the oil in a frying pan over a medium heat and cook the onion, garlic and spices for 2 minutes or until soft.

**2** Add the olives, preserved lemon and tomato, and cook for 1–2 minutes until the tomato is softened. Transfer to a bowl and add the chickpeas, then mash them until almost smooth but retaining some texture. Stir in the tahini. Season with salt and pepper to taste and scatter over the parsley to serve. Store in the refrigerator for up to 5 days.

### Brain Benefits

The flavonoids in citrus fruits such as lemons have anti-inflammatory properties that might help to ward off neurodegenerative diseases, such as Alzheimer's and Parkinson's, which are the result of the breakdown of cells in the nervous system. Including the fruits and juice in your diet can also help to boost brain function.

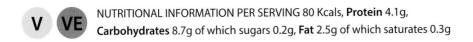

**V** **VE** NUTRITIONAL INFORMATION PER SERVING 80 Kcals, **Protein** 4.1g, **Carbohydrates** 8.7g of which sugars 0.2g, **Fat** 2.5g of which saturates 0.3g

# Garlic & Turmeric Chickpea Crunchies

**These moreish little snacks are a perfect protein pick-me-up and are an ideal alternative to popcorn or crisps/chips.**

**Serves 4**
**Preparation: 10 minutes**
**Cooking: 30 minutes**

**400g/14oz can chickpeas, drained and rinsed**
**1 tsp olive oil**
**1 tsp ground turmeric**
**½ tsp garam masala**
**½ tsp garlic salt**
**a pinch of ground black pepper**

**1** Preheat the oven to 180°C/350°F/Gas 4. Pat the chickpeas dry on paper towels and put them in a bowl.

**2** Add the oil, spices, garlic salt and pepper, and toss to coat. Arrange in a single layer on a baking sheet and cook in the oven for 30 minutes or until golden and crisp. Leave to cool, then store in an airtight container for up to 4 days.

### Brain Benefits
Chickpeas, like other pulses, are a good source of fibre which is essential for a healthy gut. They also provide iron, zinc, folate, phosphorus and B vitamins – all vital nutrients for healthy brain function.

NUTRITIONAL INFORMATION PER CRACKER 112 Kcals, **Protein** 4.2g, **Carbohydrates** 3.5g of which sugars 0.7g, **Fat** 8.4g of which saturates 0.7g

# Mixed Seeded Crackers

**For maximum nutritional benefit, these are best dehydrated using a dehydrator, but they are just as tasty baked in the oven until crisp. Use shelled hemp seeds, which have a softer texture than the whole unshelled seeds.**

**Makes 16 crackers**
**Preparation: 15 minutes**
**Cooking: 50 minutes**

150g/5½oz/1 cup whole flaxseed
60g/2¼oz/heaping ⅓ cup shelled
   hemp seeds
60g/2¼oz/scant ⅔ cup ground
   almonds
2 tomatoes, chopped
½ tsp sea salt or garlic salt
4 sun-dried tomatoes in oil, drained
juice of ½ lemon
1 tbsp nutritional yeast flakes
   (optional)
1 tsp nori flakes or sea vegetable
   flakes

**1** Preheat the oven to 170°C/325°F/Gas 3 and line a baking sheet with baking parchment. Put all the ingredients in a food processor with 2 tablespoons water and whiz until the mixture starts to come together. Scrape down the sides to make sure all the seeds are blended.

**2** Spread the mixture onto the prepared baking sheet and, using a spatula or damp hands, spread the mixture to form a rectangle about 1cm/½in thick.

**3** Mark the rectangle into 16 even crackers using the back of a blunt knife. Bake for 30 minutes or until the mixture begins to turn golden. Remove from the oven and gently flip the whole sheet over and back onto the sheet.

**4** Return to the oven and bake for a further 20 minutes or until crisp. Transfer to a wire rack to cool completely, then break into crackers. Store in an airtight container for up to 2 weeks.

**Brain Benefits**
Nori flakes added to the mix are an easy way to boost the iodine content of the crackers. Iodine is an essential mineral for brain function. Nutritional yeast flakes contain B vitamins that help to boost the production of neurotransmitters.

# INDEX

adrenal glands 37, 38
alcohol 49, 53
Alzheimer's disease 6, 8–9, 39, 41, 44
amino acids 46, 48
antioxidants 23, 35, 40–1, 55
anxiety 47
apples:
  beetroot apple kraut 68
  caramel apple pancakes 91
  creamy apple & cinnamon kale crisps 207
  fermented apple sauce 71
  squash & apple soup 106
asparagus & salmon mini frittatas 103
aubergines:
  caponata 159
  grilled lamb with aubergine 139
  roasted aubergine & kale tapenade 208
autoimmune diseases 20
avocados:
  avocado mayo 142
  lemon cheesecake layered pots 184

bacteria, in gut 29–31
banana: acai berry bowl 83
barbecue sauce, fruity 71
barbecue tempeh bowl 115
beans 16
  Mexican bean burgers 179
  pan-fried halibut with haricot beans 155
  Sicilian courgetti with olives 173
beef: satay beef skewers with pineapple 137
beetroot:
  beet chocolate brownies 195
  beetroot apple kraut 68
  beetroot kvass 64
berries:
  acai berry bowl 83
  berry chia jam 73

berry crumble mug cake 191
  chocolate berry swirl bread 199
  superberry swirl kefir ice cream 192
bibimbap, quinoa 168
black beans: Mexican bean burgers 179
bliss balls, brain protein 202
blood–brain barrier 35
blood sugar levels 8, 13, 14, 18, 22, 31
blueberries:
  blueberry & walnut granola 88
  orange blueberry muffins 193
bone broth 53, 62
brain:
  Alzheimer's disease 6, 8–9, 39, 41, 44
  blood-brain barrier 35
  effects of stress 37
  fats and 32–4
  gluten sensitivity and 20–1
  glycation 14
  gut health and 29
  homocysteine levels 9
  improving circulation 38–9
  neurotransmitters 7, 13, 14, 34, 37, 48
  plasticity 7
  re-energizing 43–9
  toxins and 23–7
bread:
  breakfast seeded bread 94–5
  chocolate berry swirl bread 199
breakfast mocha no-bake protein bars 87
breakfast seeded bread 94–5
broccoli:
  broccoli pesto 152
  broccoli pizza 171
  broccoli rice 167
  broccoli tahini cream soup 107
  cauliflower & broccoli butternut "cheese" 177

garlic broccoli, lentil & tomato salad 118
  green shakshuka 99
  roasted veggie loaf 180
broth, chicken 62
brownies, beet chocolate 195
buckwheat crunchies, chai-spiced 84
Buddha bowl, mushroom 176
bullet-proof mocha mushroom smoothie 80
burgers:
  Mexican bean burgers 179
  Thai-spiced burgers 136

cabbage:
  beetroot apple kraut 68
  coleslaw sauerkraut 67
  fruity spiced kimchi 68
  pineapple & turmeric sauerkraut 67
caffeine 49, 53
cakes:
  beet chocolate brownies 195
  green lime cream cake 196
  mug cakes 190–1
cannellini beans: Sicilian courgetti with olives 173
caramel apple pancakes 91
carbohydrates 13, 14–17, 51
cashew nuts: cinnamon nut butter cookies 200
cauliflower:
  cauliflower & broccoli butternut "cheese" 177
  cauliflower egg fried rice 172
  cauliflower rice 167
  smoky cauliflower bites 204
  speedy nori hand rolls 131
celeriac rice 167
chai-spiced buckwheat crunchies 84
"cheese", cauliflower & broccoli butternut 177

cheese:
  feta, herb & olive muffins 92
  cheese & onion kale crisps 207
chia seeds: berry chia jam 73
chicken:
  chicken broth 62
  chicken burrito bowl 127
  chicken enchilada soup 110
  chicken pad thai 143
  crispy chicken bites 142
  miso pot noodle 117
  one-pot Indian chicken 144
chickpeas:
  garlic & turmeric chickpea
    crunchies 210
  smashed lemon chickpea spread
    209
  spicy chickpea bowl 115
  spinach, chickpea & chorizo hash
    89
chilli breakfast bowl 101
chimichurri, minty 139
chocolate:
  beet chocolate brownies 195
  bullet-proof mocha mushroom
    smoothie 80
  chocolate nut spread 75
  chocolate overnight peanut
    bowl 83
  chocolate berry swirl bread 199
  mocha breakfast cake 191
  vegan chocolate peanut butter
    mug cake 191
  white chocolate macadamia
    butter 75
cholesterol 34
choline 44
chorizo: spinach, chickpea &
  chorizo hash 89
cinnamon cream peaches 187
cinnamon nut butter cookies 200
coconut: sugar-free strawberry
    butter 75
coconut milk:
  coconut yogurt 61
  golden milk turmeric smoothie
    79
  matcha coconut ice cream 188

  whipped coconut cream 72
coconut oil 34
cod: spiced fish fingers 156
coeliac disease 20–1
coffee: mocha breakfast cake 191
cognitive decline 9
coleslaw sauerkraut 67
cookies, cinnamon nut butter 200
cordyceps mushrooms 24, 45
cortisol 37, 49
courgettes:
  courgette fries 179
  Sicilian courgetti with olives 173
crackers, mixed seeded 211
cream cheese 61
crisps, kale 206–7
cucumber:
  cucumber dill pickles 69
  green lime detox shake 78
curry, Indonesian fish 166

dementia 6, 8–9
depression 46–7, 48
detoxification 23–5, 30
diabetes 6, 8, 13
docosahexaenoic acid (DHA) 32, 33
dopamine 14, 47–8
dressings 124–5
drinks 53
  beetroot kvass 64
  green lime detox shake 78
  kefir 63
  kombucha 65
  smoothies 78–80
duck, soy-braised 146

eggs:
  asparagus & salmon mini
    frittatas 103
  cauliflower egg fried rice 172
  green shakshuka 99
  Indian spiced omelette 100
eicosapentaenoic acid (EPA) 32, 33
enteric nervous system 29
environmental toxins 23–7
epinephrine 14
erythritol 19
exercise 43–4, 47, 53

fasting 55
fats 32–4
  fats to avoid 27, 51
  fructose and 18
  healthy fats 34, 41
  metabolism 16
  omega-3 fats 32–3, 34, 39, 41, 47
  saturated fats 34
fermented apple sauce 71
fermented foods 30, 41, 66–9
feta, herb & olive muffins 92
fibre 13, 17, 18, 31
fish 27, 32, 41
  spiced fish fingers 156
  sweet potato gratin fish pie 148
  see also cod, salmon etc
flavonoids 35, 40–1
folic acid 48
frappuccino, pomegranate 80
free-radicals 23, 34, 39, 40
frittatas, asparagus & salmon mini
    103
fructose 17–18
fruit 17–18, 40–1, 53
  fruit juice 18
  see also apples, berries,
    strawberries etc

gamma-hydroxybutyric acid
    (GABA) 47
garlic & turmeric chickpea
    crunchies 210
garlic broccoli, lentil & tomato salad
    118
glucose 13–14, 17
glutathione 23, 24
gluten 20–2, 51
glycaemic load (GL) 15
glycation 14
goji berries: brain protein bliss balls
    202
golden milk turmeric smoothie 79
grains 14, 16, 21, 22, 52
granola, blueberry & walnut 88
green lime cream cake 196
green lime detox shake 78
green matcha latte 79
green shakshuka 99

gummies, strawberry cream 203
gut 28–31
    fermented foods 30
    gluten and 20–1
    and inflammation 29–30
    prebiotics 30–1
gut-healing savoury blend 78

haemoglobin blood tests 14
halibut:
    Indonesian fish curry 166
    pan-fried halibut with haricot
      beans 155
haricot beans, pan-fried halibut
    with 155
hazelnuts: chocolate nut spread 75
heart disease 18, 34
high blood sugar 8, 14, 22
homocysteine 9, 34
hormones 34, 37

ice cream:
    matcha coconut ice cream 188
    superberry swirl kefir ice cream
      192
immune system 20, 23–4, 29
Indian spiced omelette 100
Indonesian fish curry 166
inflammation 7, 8, 23–4, 29–30, 32,
    35, 40, 41
insulin 8, 13, 14, 16, 31
insulin resistance 13, 16
intestinal permeability 20, 22, 29
iron 47

jam, berry chia 73
jjamppong 111

kale:
    kale crisps 206–7
    lemon & tahini wilted kale & nori
      salad 120
    meatball & kale soup 108
    roasted aubergine & kale
      tapenade 208
    super kale pesto 153
    sweet greens 82

kefir 63
    superberry swirl kefir ice cream
      192
ketchup 70
ketones 17, 34
kimchi, fruity spiced 68
kombucha 65
kvass, beetroot 64
L-acetyl carnitine 44
L-glutamine 24
L-huperzine 44
laksa, light prawn 162
lamb:
    grilled lamb with aubergine 139
    meatballs with butternut squash
      pasta 134
    Thai-spiced burgers 136
leaky gut 20, 22, 29–30
learning new skills 44
leeks: soy-braised duck with
    garlicky leeks 146
leftovers sushi bowl 116
lemon:
    lemon & tahini wilted kale & nori
      salad 120
    lemon cheesecake layered pots
      184
    smashed lemon chickpea spread
      209
lentils: garlic broccoli, lentil &
    tomato salad 118
lettuce: massaged-greens bowl 116
limes:
    green lime cream cake 196
    green lime detox shake 78
lion's mane mushrooms 45
liver 23–5, 34
low blood sugar 14
luo han guo (monk fruit) 19

maca & cinnamon-spiced protein
    mug cake 190
macadamia nuts:
    roasted macadamia tomato
      pesto 153
    white chocolate macadamia
      butter 75

maccachino kale crisps 207
mackerel:
    pomegranate-glazed mackerel
      160
    quick & spicy mackerel nasi
      goreng 164
magnesium 14, 38, 46, 47
massaged-greens bowl 116
matcha:
    green matcha latte 79
    matcha coconut ice cream 188
mayonnaise, blender 70
meatball & kale soup 108
meatballs with butternut squash
    pasta 134
Mediterranean diet 40
Mediterranean red rice salad 123
medium-chain triglycerides (MCTs)
    34
memory 43, 44
Mexican bean burgers 179
minerals 14, 40
mint & caper dressing 125
miso:
    miso pot noodle 117
    miso tahini orange dressing 125
    sweet miso vinegar kale crisps
      207
mocha breakfast cake 191
monk fruit (luo han guo) 19
monounsaturated fats 34
mood boosters 46–7
Moroccan-spiced salmon Niçoise
    129
muffins:
    feta, herb & olive muffins 92
    orange blueberry muffins 193
mug cakes, protein-boost 190–1
mushrooms 41, 45
    bullet-proof mocha mushroom
      smoothie 80
    mushroom Buddha bowl 176
    savoury waffles with creamy
      mushrooms 96
mussels, vegetable spaghetti with
    163
N-acetyl-cysteine (NAC) 24

nasi goreng 164
neurogenesis 43
neurotransmitters 7, 13, 14, 29, 34, 37, 48
nitric oxide 38–9
noodles: miso pot noodle 117
nori: speedy nori hand rolls 131
nourish bowls 114–16
nut butters 74–5
    see also cashew nuts, walnuts etc

oats:
    breakfast mocha no-bake protein bars 87
oils 33, 34
oily fish 32, 41
omega-3 fats 32–3, 34, 39, 41, 47
omelette, Indian spiced 100
one-pot Indian chicken 144
orange blueberry muffins 193
oxidative stress 39–40
oxygen 38–9

pad thai, chicken 143
Paleo diet 22
pancakes, caramel apple 91
pancreas 13
parsnip rice 167
peaches, cinnamon cream 187
peanut butter:
    chocolate overnight peanut bowl 83
    vegan chocolate peanut butter mug cake 191
peas:
    gut-healing savoury blend 78
    tartare peas 156
peppers:
    romesco sauce 158
    turmeric-spiced leftover pickles 69
pesto 151, 152–3
phenylalanine 48
phospholipid choline 44
pickles, cucumber dill 69

pineapple:
    pineapple & turmeric sauerkraut 67
    satay beef skewers with pineapple 137
pizza, broccoli 171
polypeptides 21
polyphenols 40–1
pomegranate frappuccino 80
pomegranate-glazed mackerel 160
portion sizes 16
prawns:
    light prawn laksa 162
    sweet potato gratin fish pie 148
    Vietnamese prawn salad 128
prebiotics 30–1
protein 16, 22, 52
protein bars, breakfast mocha no-bake 87
protein-boost mug cakes 190–1
pulses 16, 52
puttanesca 119

quinoa bibimbap 168

reishi mushrooms 45
rice: Mediterranean red rice salad 123
rice malt syrup 19
rices, vegetable 167
romesco sauce 158

salads:
    garlic broccoli, lentil & tomato salad 118
    lemon & tahini wilted kale & nori salad 120
    Mediterranean red rice salad 123
    Moroccan-spiced salmon Niçoise 129
    Vietnamese prawn salad 128
salmon:
    Moroccan-spiced salmon Niçoise 129
    salmon tataki 147
    see also smoked salmon
san choy bau 140

sardines with 5-minute romesco sauce 158
satay beef skewers with pineapple 137
saturated fats 34
sauces:
    fermented apple sauce 71
    fruity barbecue sauce 71
    ketchup 70
    puttanesca 119
sauerkraut:
    beetroot apple kraut 68
    coleslaw sauerkraut 67
    pineapple & turmeric sauerkraut 67
sea bass: grilled sea bass with caponata 159
sea vegetables 41
    vegetarian hot & sour soup 112
seafood: jjamppong 111
seeds: mixed seeded crackers 211
serotonin 14, 46–7
shakshuka, green 99
Sicilian courgetti with olives 173
sleep 37, 48–9
smoked salmon:
    asparagus & salmon mini frittatas 103
    hot-smoked salmon, pancetta & dill pesto tart 151
    leftovers sushi bowl 116
smoothie bowls 82–3
smoothies 78–80
snacks 54
soups:
    broccoli tahini cream soup 107
    chicken enchilada soup 110
    jjamppong 111
    meatball & kale soup 108
    squash & apple soup 106
    vegetarian hot & sour soup 112
soy-braised duck 146
spices 52
spinach, chickpea & chorizo hash 89
squash:
    cauliflower & broccoli butternut "cheese" 177

meatballs with butternut squash
pasta 134
roasted veggie loaf 180
squash & apple soup 106
stevia 19
strawberries:
strawberry cream gummies 203
sugar-free strawberry butter 75
stress 37–8
sugar 13–19, 51
super-green herb dressing 124
superberry swirl kefir ice cream 192
supplements 33, 37, 38, 44, 47, 48
sushi bowl 116
sweet greens 82
sweet potatoes:
hot-smoked salmon, pancetta &
dill pesto tart 151
sweet potato gratin fish pie 148
sweeteners 19, 53

tacos, sticky orange tempeh 175
tapenade, roasted aubergine &
kale 208
tarts: hot-smoked salmon, pancetta
& dill pesto tart 151
tea:
chai-spiced buckwheat
crunchies 84
green matcha latte 79
kombucha 65
matcha coconut ice cream 188

tempeh:
barbecue tempeh bowl 115
sticky orange tempeh tacos 175
vegetarian hot & sour soup 112
Thai-spiced burgers 136
tomatoes:
chilli breakfast bowl 101
fruity barbecue sauce 71
ketchup 70
roasted macadamia tomato
pesto 153
spicy tomato kale crisps 207
vegetable ribbons with
puttanesca 119
toxins 23–7, 30, 35
triglycerides 18
tryptophan 46, 49
turkey:
chilli breakfast bowl 101
meatball & kale soup 108
san choy bau 140
turmeric:
garlic & turmeric chickpea
crunchies 210
golden milk turmeric smoothie
79
pineapple & turmeric sauerkraut
67
turmeric-spiced leftover pickles
69

vegan diet 22, 48

vegetables 15, 16, 40–1, 52
fermented vegetables 66–9
turmeric-spiced leftover pickles
69
vegetable ribbons with
puttanesca 119
vegetable rices 167
vegetable spaghetti with
mussels 163
see also peppers, tomatoes etc
vegetarian hot & sour soup 112
veggie loaf, roasted 180
Vietnamese prawn salad 128
vitamins 14, 32, 40
vitamin B complex 9, 14, 30, 38,
44, 46
vitamin C 38
vitamin K2 30

waffles: savoury waffles with
creamy mushrooms 96
walnuts: blueberry & walnut
granola 88
weight loss 15
whey 61

xylitol 19

yacon syrup 19
yogurt 60–1

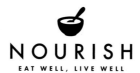

# NOURISH
#### EAT WELL, LIVE WELL

Here at Nourish we're all about wellbeing through food and drink – irresistible dishes with
a serious good-for-you factor. If you want to eat and drink delicious things that set you up for
the day, suit any special diets, keep you healthy and make the most of the ingredients you have,
we've got some great ideas to share with you. Come over to our blog for wholesome recipes
and fresh inspiration – nourishbooks.com